# Stroke Victor™
## How to Go from Stroke Victim to Stroke Victor

# STROKE VICTOR
## How to Go from Stroke Victim to Stroke Victor
**© 2014 Robert Mandell - All Rights Reserved**

**For Information Contact:**

**Creative Projects International Ltd.**
4001 Santa Barbara Blvd.
Naples, FL 34104

Info@creativeprojintl.com

# STROKE VICTOR™
ISBN: 978-0-9818222-7-3

Library of Congress: 2014943314

# PRAISE FOR *"STROKE VICTOR"* IN THE HEALTHCARE COMMUNITY

"Mandell brings a new and refreshing focus on recovery after a stroke. He shows how he was able to take control of his recovery after a devastating stroke and mixes humor, determination and a positive attitude in this inspiring book."

Dr. Justin C. McArthur
Director, Department of Neurology
Johns Hopkins University School of Medicine

"I applaud Bob for writing this book from the patient's perspective! He sends a strong message about the importance of self-advocacy, determination, and participation in research."

Cindy Drapal, MSN, MHA, RN, NEA-BC
Director, Neuroscience Institute
Lee Memorial Health System

"In this intensely honest view of the challenges of overcoming stroke, Bob relates not only the 'how to' but also the 'why' in this incredibly hope-filled book. This is a much needed resource not only for the potential 'Stroke Victor' but also for the caregiver!"

Mollie Venglar DSc, MSPT, NCS
Florida Gulf Coast University
Department of Rehabilitation Sciences

"To my knowledge there are several great textbooks on neuropsychological rehabilitation for professionals available. Bob's book though fills a wide open gap for people afflicted with almost any type of TBI, but strokes in particular. It is my belief that it will be tremendously helpful and encouraging to the many unfortunate victims suffering the same or similar physiological and psychological consequences Bob so successfully overcame. In addition, I support Bob in establishing a stroke research foundation to further our understanding about this often overlooked cause of death and disability which impacts so many individuals."

Udo Fischer PhD LMHC, Dipl. Psych

"Bob Mandell has written an important book, *Stroke Victor*. At the core of his book is the mantra for every stroke victim to be positive, always make your maximum effort, never give up, don't focus on your deficits, celebrate every improvement in function, if you fail, try harder to achieve, set reasonable goals and continue therapy and rehabilitation on a daily basis, forever. He also emphasizes that you have to build a team to support and assist you in your efforts, an area he discusses in the book.

*Stroke Victor* makes the point that patients should be open to trying alternative methods of therapy that have not been accepted and evaluated in the mainstream of stroke rehabilitation, since he has benefited from many of them. In addition, I believe in his emphasis on being brave and trying to return to function in the community and not be inhibited by the social impact of your disability. Understand that people will be helpful and make accommodations to meet your needs. Plan to participate in more activities to increase the quality of your life.

This is an excellent read for other stroke victims, their families, friends and supporters. Going by chapter he describes his experiences in the various steps in his journey from the acute hospital to inpatient physical, speech, occupational therapy, to home. Then his participation in the continuum of his multi-modality rehabilitation therapy in an out- patient setting and then many years of continued participation in other forms of therapy. He describes accurately, offering practical recommendations for participation in the activities of daily living.

His Odyssey has motivated him to become a counselor, mentor and advocate for patients who suffer the variable disabilities secondary to stroke. At this time, Bob is committed to launching a research foundation with its mission to advance discoveries that will be helpful in the prevention, improved treatment and recovery from strokes, as well as the development of new modalities of rehabilitation."

William D. Ertag MD, FAAN

"This is an easy to read book and will be a helpful tool to both family and friends of loved ones who have suffered the life-changing effects of a stroke. Mr. Mandell's story should be shared as it is one that can be an example of hope. I believe a lot of good will come to those who read this!"

Michael Legal
CEO – First Alternatives, LLC

"Bob's story expands our thinking on stroke recovery! His exploration of innovative therapies which go beyond prescribed intense rehabilitation inspires hope and limitless possibilities."

Mary Bonnette, PhD – Stroke Caregiver/Family Member

## PRAISE FOR *"STROKE VICTOR"* IN THE PATIENT/CAREGIVER COMMUNITY

"Bob's new book, *Stroke Victor* is a compendium of great advice on what stroke victims should investigate and do to enrich their lives and speed them along on their road to recovery. Bob is the "new face" and champion for stroke victims today. His founding of The Stroke Research Foundation shows his dedication to improving the quality of post-stroke lifestyles for all victims and their families. I urge every stroke victim and family to read this book and become involved in Bob's Foundation. Your freedom is waiting."

Mike Burns
CEO – A+ Conferencing, Stroke Caregiver/Family Member

"I have now read *Stoke Victor* three times. It is an amazing book. It is strong medicine for stroke victims and can be of great help to them. This book should be available at every rehab facility to show stroke victims and their caregivers the journey to a quality life after suffering a stroke. They must keep reaching! I wish I had this knowledge when my dearest aunt/godmother suffered her stroke."

Mary Kay Lane – Stroke Caregiver/Family Member

"Because of reading Bob's book, I do feel I can go through a nasty course of cancer radiation treatments. It is his book and the sayings that I think about while I am getting the treatment. I really like the pictures and quotes at the beginning of each section."

Judith Goke - Cancer Survivor

"Mr. Mandell has added remarkably important thinking to the process of stroke recovery. By learning from his experiences and holistic thinking, victims and their caregivers can measurably improve their lives."

Bob Jones - Retired Advertising Executive, Entrepreneur and Friend too many Stroke Victims

"This is truly a book for anyone who is or knows someone recovering from a stroke. You went above and beyond to provide a very deep holistic and realistic view of how one can educate themselves on all options available including traditional health care, alternative services, nutrition and mindset. This book is needed and must get in the hands of everyone - even those not touched by stroke, because the principals in this book truly empower a patient and their caregivers to go beyond the basics and get the very best support and treatments. This book will serve masses!!"

Dena Moscola - Leadership Coach, Consultant and Stroke Supporter

# ABOUT AUTHOR BOB – WHAT'S UP!

## STROKE COACHING SERVICE

Understanding the sudden AND possibly overwhelming situation you, the survivor, and/or you, the caregiver partner may find yourself encountering, we have started a **Stroke Coaching Service** to assist post-stroke families.

The services can be provided in person and/or through our Tele-Medicine service, which allows for the family to participate from the comfort of their home.

The Coaching service is a family customized service which includes some, or all, of the following depending on need:
- assistance in advocating for patient needs;
- identifying appropriate and sometimes difficult to find recovery resources;
- help in the creation of a stroke recovery plan, and then, coaching in the execution of the plan;
- navigating the clinical research world (if there is an interest);
- assistance and support to the caregiver partner;
- providing motivational support, and
- being a sympathetic and supportive ear from a couple who "have walked the walk".

## SPEAKING ENGAGEMENTS

Now that I am able to speak publicly once again, I conduct **motivational speaking engagements** focused on a balanced, holistic and comprehensive approach to personal and corporate growth, drawing on my experiences becoming a Stroke Victor and a successful and varied business career.

**A portion of the proceeds from these endeavors will be donated to The Stroke Research Foundation,** an advocacy and research funding initiative which is discussed in the Afterword section of the book.

By way of background, I received my MS Degree in Business from Penn State and a BBA Degree from Pace University in New York.

Previous to my stroke, I was a corporate executive, a partner in an international management consulting firm, an Adjunct Instructor at Fairfield University and an entrepreneur.

I may be contacted directly at Bob@StrokeVictor.com.

This book is dedicated to my wife, Debbie.
Without her unvarnished support I would not be where I am today.

I Love You!

# TABLE OF CONTENTS

# ACKNOWLEDGEMENTS

This project began one February, 2013 day in the home office of my good friend, Dr. Bill Colburn, retired distinguished Professor of Communications, University of Michigan, and a former owner of a speakers' bureau in Ann Arbor, MI. I take this professional communicator very seriously when he suggests something.

*"Bob, you have to talk about this! You and Debbie just got back from six weeks of traveling in Australia and New Zealand. You weren't even on a tour. Here you are, a massive stroke survivor, and traveling around the world. You have to tell people, other stroke survivors and folks with other disabilities. They will be inspired! They will see how they can do it also."*

So began a personal journey, something I had avoided doing for all of these years. Looking back to write this book!

Let me say at the outset that the book is not just about me or us. Far from it! It's really about the many sung and unsung people who have helped me get to the place where I once again have the mental and speaking capacity and the energy to write and speak about this book.

It's about the folks at Main Street Rehab in Danbury, Connecticut, in 1996 through 1998, particularly Kathie White and Carrie who initially helped me to build a base from which I could grow and excel; it's about the team at the Brain Rehabilitation Center in Gainesville, Florida, where I made considerable progress participating in their clinical research; it's about my dear friend, physical therapist Irene Hujsa in Bonita Springs, Florida, who tirelessly researched my case at night and then exposed me to the many innovative therapies that have made a remarkable difference; it's about a new friend, Dr. Mary Bonnette, who is now helping me with my balance issues, and it's about my business partner, Andy Jacobs who kept our startup company growing while keeping the money spigot flowing.

Udo Fisher, PhD in Naples, FL was instrumental in the development of the chapters on depression and for that, and his friendship, I am most grateful.

I have been fortunate to have been in two writing groups in Naples, Fl. Both contributed to improving my writing skills for which I thank the members.

Last, but definitely not least, my family and friends who supported me in one way or another throughout my recovery, and the book writing.

To all, I say a heart-felt and humble **THANK YOU**.

I have tried to write this book in the minute, to recreate the story and the lessons as they unfolded, however I am a first-time author, not a professional writer. To that end, I have been fortunate to find a publisher willing to bet on me. For that I thank, Michael Baumohl. He is educating me on the realities of book publishing in this digital age.

Let's set some expectations. **This book is meant to be a "How-To" book, not a memoir,** as Michael was very clear at the beginning that he would not publish a memoir. *"Memoirs do not sell unless you are Bill or Hillary Clinton or in their league."*

***"What you are describing to me is a very important "how-to" book that, I and many others, will be very interested in."*** As such, the book is how get on with your life after a disabling disease like a stroke, even if, at the end of the day some deficits remain, as they have with me.

To give the book some breath, personality and hopefully make it come alive, I have used my, and our stories and experiences to best convey the messages and lessons. For these reasons in writing the book, I was not especially focused on the time-line of my recovery.

However, even a casual consideration of a time-line results in an important message of this book which continues to this very day:

There has been a **constant search for new recovery opportunities!**

After we moved to Florida in early 2002, and having experienced a several year plateau in Connecticut at what I considered an unsatisfactory level, I became more inquisitive, self-advocating and ultimately happened upon some newer traditional therapies and excellent therapists, several little known integrative approaches, and was introduced to the potential benefits of participating in clinical research in a study subject role. The sum of these made a remarkable difference in my recovery as we will together explore."

*I pray this book and the shared lessons are helpful! Enjoy!*

# RELEASE

*I have to go on record!*

**The views expressed in this book are my own, not medical advice.**

I have written this book based on my, our perspectives and experiences. I am not a physician or clinician of any kind and make no representations in any way in that regard.

There is no assurance that what worked for me will work for anyone else and I take no responsibility, financial or any otherwise in that regard. Every person is different. Every stroke or disability is different.

The reader acknowledges and accepts that, I, we, make no promises of any kind and that Robert (Bob) and Deborah Mandell, Stroke Victor, SV Media Group, LLC. and its officers, shareholders, employees, agents, successors or assigns make no promise, representation or guarantee of any kind whatsoever other than that specifically specified, without limitation, concerning a reader's progress as a result of reading this book or following any of the techniques that have been described or used.

You further acknowledge that any evaluation, expression or comment that the author or anyone mentioned in the book has made, or may have made, now or in the future, is an expression of opinion only and in no way constitutes a representation, guarantee or promise of any kind.

*Sorry, but this is the world we live in!*

*Additional Note:* Recovering from Stroke is "no walk in the park". One thing it is – it is emotional, and though doable, it is tough. As such, in various sections of the book, I use slang words to reflect my emotions at the time.

If anyone is offended, I apologize but this is the way it was!

# FOREWORD

I have known and admired Bob Mandell for years, both as my friend and my patient. A businessman by training and nature, Bob has taken firm control of his recovery from a devastating stroke. Like an entrepreneur starting a new venture, Bob has done his research, vetted the key players involved in his care and is not afraid to explore new ideas that can yield great dividends in increased quality of life.

I am so glad that Bob has now chosen to share his experiences with the public. *Stroke Victor* will save you time, give you comfort and, perhaps most importantly, **reassure you that you are not alone in your struggle.** You will learn a great deal from Bob's book. *Stroke Victor* that will help guide you to the right types of facilities, programs that have benefitted him the most and getting on with your life.

On a personal level, I was thrilled to read how Bob benefitted from the non-traditional techniques that I often incorporate into my practice. As Bob tells us, **don't be afraid to try something new. Do not settle for the status quo.** Not all techniques will work for everyone, but follow Bob's lead and never give up looking for the care that works best for you. I have had so many patients who could be helped by this book.

Bob has learned a valuable lesson that everyone would do well to remember: **in the end, only you can really be responsible for your care.** Even if you aren't as lucky as Bob to have a partner as dedicated and capable as his wife Debbie, Bob's example can help you cope with the immediate aftermath of your stroke and then your re-entry into the world.

From mastering an elevator, to romancing your partner, and to traveling around the world, *Stroke Victor* will be an indispensable guide to your life after stroke.

**IRENE U. HUJSA, PT.**
**3/20/2015**

# PROLOGUE

It's June 2014. I've been honored by an invitation from the Canadian Partnership for Stroke Recovery to attend their annual convention in Ottawa, Canada as a media person. This was to be the first public initiative of my new career as author, advocate, speaker and media person focusing on stroke, the disease, and particularly stroke recovery, something I have become intimately familiar with.

Frankly, I was somewhat nervous being a media person, as that was out of my comfort zone, though I am now changing that. (New opportunities, new horizons!) Arriving early, I was quickly met by the Partnership's Communications Director, Cathy Campbell. Gracious as she was, she got me sorted out with brochures, printed materials, my badge and cap.

As I was walking towards the meeting room which would serve several hundred scientists one of the participants spotted me in my newly minted logo shirt – *Stroke Victor*. Looking directly at me, he said of the shirt, "BOLD!"

Taken aback, I smiled and quietly said, "Yes" as we proceeded in different directions. Reflecting back, I should have said, not so quietly,

***"Yes, that's right. BOLD is good and BOLD is what's needed when you have had a stroke and want to recover."*** I made a mental note to have that response at my ready should a similar situation again present itself.

Thinking back,

*Nineteen years ago when I had my stroke, I definitely wasn't thinking Bold.* And I don't think that I was the exception. Actually I wasn't thinking very much at all, or for that matter, speaking or anything else. I couldn't! I had been hit by a massive brain attack and was reflexively responding to a monstrous problem.

Writing this book, **I realized that how one responds, either reflexively, by design, cajoling, by sheer will power, or, not at all, will substantially impact how yours and your caregiver's future lives will go.** That's the reality, and in some cases, the sad reality! But I am here to tell you…

**WE CAN ALL BE STROKE VICTORS - WE CAN ALL DO IT!**

**And with that…on that cold, gray and dank late January night, new lives began…**

# Part I

## *Darkness Descends*

With so many seconds lost
the sky
becomes pitch black!

*- Bob Mandell*

*"Hope is stronger than despair."*

Cardinal Timothy Dolan – 4/20/2014

# CHAPTER 1
# ADVICE - WHAT ADVICE?

The year is 1996, and changes are coming that are…

**"Mr. Mandell, you should think about accommodating a future life in a wheelchair, as you are now,"** the unsympathetic doctor with really bad bedside manners said.

At the ripe young age of 53, and recently moved into a Stamford, Connecticut, nursing home that's the advice I got from the home's attending physician,

***Fuck You.*** *Fuck You!* I thought but couldn't say. There weren't words, even with my then limited intellectual capacity.

**"With strokes you get the great majority of your recovery during the first year, and you are in pretty bad shape,"** the doctor continued.

*I thought. A year's a long time—that's plenty of time to beat this,* but I was in total shock from the doctor's words, nonetheless.

*There's no way. What do you know? No way!*

When my wife of 18 months, Debbie, heard it, she thought the same and more. "I didn't wait nearly 25 years for the right man to have this happen and not beat it."

*But wait, maybe, maybe he is right!*

A lovely young speech therapist gave me a three-word sentence to repeat as she was evaluating me. I think it was "*I love you.*"

I couldn't repeat it!

I tried a few more times. Imagine me who could always speak? A former management consultant! Heck, management consultants talk in their sleep!

Now, for the first time, almost three weeks in, I thought, I must be sicker than I realize. And did I mention that I was still unable to control my bowels or go to the bathroom unattended?

*Holy Shit! I am much sicker than I thought! This could be much more serious.*

*Could the nasty doctor be right?*

# CHAPTER 2
# SHOCK AND AWE

On that dreary, dank and cold January early evening in Ridgefield, Connecticut, I had gone to bed on the top floor of our triplex townhouse. As I went home from work, I had gone to the doctor who said I had flu symptoms. I had a terrible headache and generally felt lousy which was a rarity for high-energy me. But that headache, wow!

*I never felt anything like this before.*

Debbie was teaching her women's Adult Education exercise class in Greenwich, CT so she would not be home until 9 p.m. I was alone in bed and fitfully sleeping.

Suddenly, I felt something snap in my head. My headache was worse.

*What's happened? What's happened to me? My God! I can't move my right leg. I can't move it! Wait. My right hand isn't moving either. What the hell!*

I pulled at my right hand with my left hand but it was hanging uselessly.

*Wait, my right side isn't moving. Let's see – take it easy now. The left's ok –that's good. I'm scared. What the hell. Where's Debbie? When is she going to be home? Not for a while.*

I looked at the clock on the TV.

*It's too early. I can hardly move. Something serious has happened.*

*Call 911! But the house is locked up. They're going to have to knock the door down. No, no, I don't want that – what a mess!*

*I think I've had a stroke. What else could it be? It must be a stroke.*

*I can't sit up in bed – try – try again. Better call 911. I'm paralyzed – no my right side is, but I can't reach the phone next to me.*

The phone was on the night stand directly next to the bed on my right. Too far!

*Come on – reach!*

My right side was not moving so I couldn't reach around as I normally would.

*Call 911! Come on. Push, push, and roll over. Turn around. Roll over. I can't. I can't. Come on. Reach it with your left hand. Stretch – roll over.*

*There I've got it. Damn, I dropped the phone. Come on, for Christ's sake!*

*Take it easy now. Slow down – pick up the phone.*

Luckily the phone didn't fall to the floor, just on to the bed next to me

*Come on, dial 911.*

"Hello, I think I have had a stroke. 120-18 Prospect Street. Mandell, Bob. Don't come—my wife's not home. Our house is locked up. We'll call you when my wife gets home.

**And believe it or not the operator listened to me**--and didn't send help. She didn't send help for a disease where every second, every minute is critical.

But wait – my crazy irrationality gets even better!

*Maybe I should go downstairs –I can't get up. I can't walk. How do I*

*do this? I can hardly move. I'm paralyzed – no, just on my right side. I'm confused.*

*Yes, better go down –I guess they're going to take me to the hospital. I'll make it easier for them – don't want a mess. My head hurts – my right side is not moving much. Shit. But how do I do this?*

It wasn't that far to the stairs, maybe six or seven feet.

*Can't get up – can't sit up.*

*Ok, take it easy – just roll over and get to the floor. Easy now, slide down! There, I'm on the floor leaning against the bed.*

*Roll over. Now, just roll to the stairs, grab the base of the bureau to help – got it. I'm almost there – come on. Pull myself. Grab the furniture leg – keep rolling. It's not that far – pull yourself along the carpet.*

I pulled myself to the stairs.

*I'll just grab the banister and hold on and slip down one step at a time.*

*It looks so far down – Shit! What am I doing? Quick, grab the banister! My God – I'm rolling. I'm rolling down the stairs. Grab on –quick. I can't. Damn, I missed it.*

I landed on the wooden floor in the living room sprawled out immobile, and must have passed out for a few hours until Debbie opened the garage door under me.

At the sound of the garage door opening, I awoke…

Debbie was home.

"Quick, get up here. Hurry up." "I'm coming. Take it easy," she shouted from the garage.

It was nearly 9 p.m. and she was starved, thinking that I had dinner ready as I normally did when she taught her class and I was home.

"I think I've had a stroke. Quick—call 911."

I still was able to speak, but it was getting garbled, Debbie told me later.

Calling 911 in smallish Ridgefield, she got the same operator I had spoken with earlier.

"You're home Mrs. Mandell! Your husband called and said he thought he was having a stroke but not to come - so we didn't."

"**WHAT?** Are you kidding?" she screamed to the operator.

"We'll be right there."

⌂

The ambulance was here.

"Are you taking him to Danbury Hospital?"

Yes, the driver indicated. "I'll go with him in the ambulance," Debbie said. "No, Mrs. Mandell, better you follow us so you have a way to get home. Just stay with us."

By now, my speech was gone and I had passed out again. I don't remember being taken down to the ambulance or into the hospital, nor are there any memories of being examined or being taken to surgery. None!

Stunned as she was, Debbie called good friends, Mary Kay and Glenn, who lived just across the street.

The ambulance took me to Danbury with Debbie following right behind. Now, fairly late into the night, our friends also went to the hospital to support her and see if there was anything they could do. Debbie was there most of the night.

◌

The next day I awoke groggily and tried unsuccessfully to sit up in bed. Debbie said a neurologist had performed surgery during the night on the back of my head where I had suffered a brain bleed, a hemorrhagic stroke.

I could not sit up in bed by myself. Though I was struggling, I could not sit up on my own! My right arm was hanging uselessly so I tried to lift myself up on my left elbow as I became more awake.

It was not happening. I was paralyzed on my entire right side from head to toe. My neck hurt and was stiff. I was having trouble moving my head from side to side.

But that wasn't the half of it.

*Let's see just how bad it is.*

I had lost all feeling on my right side except for some annoying tingling in my right limbs. The sensation was almost as if someone was using little needles on my skin. I took my left hand and moved it from the left side of my stomach to the right to see if and where my feeling changed. About midway across my stomach all feeling disappeared as if someone had drawn a line down my body and given me a shot of Novocain. Unfortunately, my penis was on the numb side!

*Is that a diaper I feel?*

I was incontinent, and all of my other plumbing seemed to be gone. I wasn't able to say very much and what did get out was garbled. Because I didn't have a mirror, I wasn't aware that my face was seriously contorted, something called facial droop. It was hanging down on the right side while I drooled onto the towel that was on my chest. Debbie had had the movable mirrors removed so I couldn't see myself. That was probably a darn good idea!

○

To top it off, a severe case of hiccups had developed which the doctors were unable to control, so, I mostly slept out of exhaustion! My time – about ten days-- in the hospital is mostly a blur with a few people visiting and doctors coming and going. It's all pretty vague. My former wife, Lorraine visited, as did my business partner, Andy. I guess some others came to see me also.

My two children, Amy and David, were very concerned and wanted to come home to see me. It didn't seem like they could do much and it would have been very expensive. We decided that they should stay put at college in Pennsylvania and Florida and keep up with their studies.

Was it right – was it wrong – in retrospect, it was dumb and insensitive! Debbie and I were in denial about the seriousness of the situation. It was a chaotic time!

As a practical matter, the kids probably didn't study very much anyway. They were in constant telephone communication, mostly through their mother and Debbie. Yes, they probably should have come home for a short visit to see me, but since I was in such bad shape, I doubt they would have been at all reassured. Also, we didn't want them falling behind in school, particularly given the amount we were spending on their education.

○

The good news -- and it certainly was good news -- I had survived a massive stroke. **I had survived!** Given my stroke's intensity, it could have killed me like these brain attacks do to so many others.

*That said, none of this was good. Not good at all!*

Thinking back, I doubt Debbie bargained for this just eighteen months before when she happily said, "I do, in sickness and in health" on a sunny June, Sunday afternoon in tony New Canaan, Connecticut.

There we were, with smiles, among family and friends at the Roger Sherman Inn, a landmark New England country inn with a wonderful restaurant and period lodging rooms.

Debbie's comment – *I think it is worth reflecting back to when we met about 18 months before that June 1994 day in New Canaan. I spent many nights thinking about it while Bob was in the hospital and nursing home.*

*I answered his personal ad in the Greenwich Time. This was a while ago and there was no Match.com in those days. Those ads, in a column called, The Meeting Place, were a 900 telephone service in which you paid by the minute to listen to each other's short messages. Bob ran his ad for free. He also made a tape for interested woman to listen to. If you liked the ad, you could listen to the tape. It mentioned two children, being a gourmet cook, being Jewish and marriage minded, among other things. I thought to myself – that's the man for me. He cooked... Responding with a short message of my own which he listened to, I guess he liked what he heard. Meanwhile the cash register was running!*

*I was meeting quite a number of gentlemen that way, but none really had clicked. Being 45, I wanted to get married so I only answered men who indicated that they were open to marriage. I had been single for over twenty years and had all the singles relationships I cared for.*

*Amazingly, when I listened to Bob's recording, I knew who he was. I couldn't believe it. What a coincidence, but at first I didn't tell him. He had been my adjunct professor way back in 1976 when I was taking a few business courses at night at Fairfield University. He was married and had two baby children. I remembered him in a three piece suit, fatter, shorter and with the start of balding hair. I wasn't attracted to him at all!*

*But now his voice was so nice on the phone that I thought - what the heck – it's only an hour. We met for a cappuccino on a rainy late afternoon after school at Brett's Restaurant in Greenwich. Bob was planning to take his son David out for dinner as he did on Wednesdays or Thursdays. I had plans to meet some friends for a birthday party so we both knew that we were not having dinner together.*

*When Bob walked in to the restaurant with his long black cashmere coat and brownish hat, I was stunned and frankly, surprisingly, interested. We chatted for a while, he mentioned that he had taught but I still didn't let on. When we were leaving he said he would call. We've all heard that more than once! It was pouring out so that was it.*

*Well, he was serious since he called that night and we arranged to have dinner the following evening in a local Italian Restaurant, coincidentally, that we both knew, and liked. We had several dinners over the next week or two and soon it came time for Bob to pick me up at my place one Saturday evening. As I started to give him the address and directions to my coop apartment, he laughed, saying that he knew the directions. I was momentarily puzzled; it turned out that he had lived in the same apartment building with his parent's years before, after they had moved out of The Bronx.*

*Another weird coincidence I thought! This is the New York suburbs, how many thousands of buildings are there? After those several dinners, things started moving faster! But at one point, I suddenly got cold feet. Was I really ready for a big time relationship, I asked myself? Was I?*

*My cold feet warmed, so one day a few weeks later during my Winter break, I marched right into Bob's office unexpected, and the rest is history!"*

# CHAPTER 3
# PICKING MY HOME AWAY FROM HOME

"We've done all we can for your husband, Mrs. Mandell."

Without warning, and after about ten days in Danbury Hospital, Debbie heard those words. And with these words the hospital was contemplating releasing me to the unknown. And so, she had less than forty eight hours to find a facility for me!

*I have to find the right place for him fast, thought Debbie. I just have a day to do all of this. What's in Fairfield County that's any good? What about Westchester?*

Debbie got in gear. In retrospect, I think she did two very smart things:

First, she made a list of criteria she would use as she visited the seven facilities she looked at, and,

Second, she gave some thought to the kind of set up where I would excel rather than just exist!

*It's either a nursing home or he will be isolated. That will not fly with me or Bob*, she thought. (In those years, the only live-in rehabilitation center in Connecticut was at the other end of the State.)

*But a nursing home… at his age!*

Debbie thought I was too young for a nursing home but there weren't any alternatives that remotely met her criteria. As for me, I was mostly sleeping and unaware of Debbie's progress on the facilities or the hiccups.

So in February, 1996, at the ripe young age of 53 – I was to be moved to Mediplex in Stamford Connecticut, (now Long Ridge Long Term Care), a nursing home with a rehab unit that Debbie had picked from the seven she had visited.

*Stop the hiccups or let me die, I thought!*

Funny how these things happen - one day just before my transfer Debbie was speaking with an aide who told her a story of a relative who used an "out of the box" drug solution to get rid of their hiccups. Darned if we know what it was.

*"What do you mean you can't get it?"*

Amazingly, the hospital couldn't or wouldn't get the medicine! She never understood that.

Leaving the hospital in an ambulance to go to Mediplex, I fell asleep during the nearly one hour drive from Danbury to Stamford. As soon as I arrived at Mediplex, they were able to procure the medicine.

*Voila! The hiccups are gone.*

Debbie commented, *"I chose what I thought would work best for our Bob and our situation. **I prayed I was right!**"*

# CHAPTER 4
# A NURSING HOME AT 53

The then modern Mediplex (now called Long Ridge of Stamford) nursing home, where I was to live for the next three months, was located about a mile from the Merritt Parkway in Stamford. The nicely landscaped red-brick home housed about 120 residents on three levels.

At the entrance to Mediplex, to the right in front of the home, a three-foot high stone wall surrounded a bare concrete terrace. There, the aides took patients "to air" and, in nice weather visitors often sat with the residents. In the spring, the staff brought out tables and chairs so people could sit and talk. But in the winter the terrace was bare as it was a fairly windy spot on the side of a gentle hill.

When I arrived, the February weather was typical Connecticut, gray and cold. For some reason I found solace on the outdoor terrace in the front of the Home, even in the winter chill. Since my right hand was useless, an aide had to take me out and bring me back. *If the weather was clear when my therapy was over for the day, I sat there contemplating God knows what!*

Sitting alone on the terrace watching the cars and the world go by, I began to feel the weight of the realization that I was so sick that I was in a nursing home. **At 53!** I thought to myself that the other patients seemed either so much older, which obviously many of them were, or so much sicker. *Who was I kidding? There's that denial!*

Looking back it would be more than fair to say that we were in crisis. Early in our new telemarketing venture in Nebraska, for me, that was now on hold. Two kids in college with bills to pay. And a new wife who never would have imagined anything like this so soon after being married. There we were!

*Though Debbie was determined that I recover, would I have the strength? Could I physically and mentally do it?* I was not used to being sick, having never been seriously ill before. The only surgery in my history to that point was a tonsillectomy at four years of age. *Therefore untested, this was damn serious!*

*Now I had to get on with it, putting the doubts and hesitations aside.* Debbie was no nonsense, this was getting solved! I, for my part, began to adjust to life in a nursing home and more importantly, to getting better.

Still exhausted and in a fog from the now ended hiccups, Debbie and the Administrator had agreed that I would move to a private room when one became available, as it soon did. And so I was moved to a private room with a phone in this pre - mobile phone era.

A physical therapist came to my room every morning before breakfast to manually exercise my right leg, shoulder and arm to try to mitigate the paralysis. My entire shoulder area was frozen but my leg had some mobility, though I couldn't control it.

Big time rehabilitation began soon when an attendant wheeled me down to the sizable rehab room for a complete evaluation.

*This is scary – who are all of these people – this isn't private – I have to share a mat - everyone can see – I don't like this!* I met what would turn out to be my initial therapy team.

*What could I move – what wouldn't …Damn little moved, at least on my right side.*

Sitting me at a table, they gave me a pencil and paper and asked me to write something. *With my normal right-sided writing hand, I could only scribble like a baby.*

And my speech, *pretty halting, but I thought it was improving…what do I know?*

A treatment plan was soon established which called for a rigorous five-day schedule and included physical, occupational and speech therapy, each for one to two hours each per day. I also had a few Saturday morning sessions.

*This is looking pretty hard and doesn't look like much fun with all of these strange people! What's going on?*

Food is always important but this was awful. I ate their cereal for breakfast. Cheerios and milk, some toast or English muffins, all of which is really hard to ruin. At lunch, the kitchen wanted to serve me their garbage food so at one point, I visited the cooks to complain, being pushed by an aide. I still couldn't talk too much, but they understood. Debbie intervened. The kitchen staff agreed to prepare a cottage cheese and fruit salad every day. Solved!

Dinner was worse. I love macaroni and cheese so I tried their rendition once and it was absolutely awful. Can't make that – can't make anything!

*Ruthie, Debbie's mother to the rescue!*

Debbie's family lived in Stamford. So Ruthie prepared something for me, often goulash, which would last a few days. Debbie's son, Keith, or her brothers would deliver it when Debbie couldn't. On Fridays, Debbie brought in pizza or Chinese food.

*Debbie had married the cook but he was either at therapy, in bed laying uselessly, or sitting solemnly on a cold terrace at a nursing home!*

# Part II

# *A Glimmer Of Hope*

The sky is dark and foreboding
but is that a speck of light
among the clouds!

*- Bob Mandell*

# CHAPTER 5

# NOW, LET'S GET GOING!

*Therapy kept me busy.*

Since we lived in a three-level townhouse, the physical therapists were very concerned not only with my ability to walk on a flat surface but with my stair-climbing abilities. I was still in a wheelchair.

*About a month after the stroke, I took my first step - halting, with a therapist holding on, but a step.*

Every rehab session found me exercising and relearning how to walk between two parallel bars. Initially I was partially supported by a therapist. After several weeks, I could walk to the other end of the parallel bars unaided. Then, I graduated to walking outside of the bars, just using one for support. Eventually no bars were required. I started down the long hallway, at first, with a harness held by the therapist or with a quad cane, but unaided. The harness is a cloth belt the PTs put around my waist for safety. They would hold on to it so that I wouldn't fall.

The quad cane is a type of cane that has a base at the bottom and four little legs, and is designed so it can be placed on the floor in a standing position. I always preferred this type of cane because it stood on its own. (Now, there are some newer quad cane designs which are improved, one has three feet, the HurryCane®, for example, which is also worthy of consideration). In contrast, I always disliked the single pole cane. I was always worried about it falling so I was never comfortable using it. For me, single canes are a pain and I resist them to this day! It seems as though the newer canes solve this.

While I was relearning to walk unaided, the therapists very gradually started to teach me stair walking, literally one-step-at-a-time. I had to retrain my right leg that didn't want to move to do the stairs. Repetitive leg exercises got the leg going, if unsteadily.

Interestingly, most healthy people, including me in my pre – stroke state, always found going down a flight of stairs to be easier. Handicapped, I found going up much better.

Today, I still find it far easier to walk up hills and stairs, partly due to my challenged balance. When I look down a hill or a flight of stairs it is visually scary, particularly the first time. And now I find going down to be harder on the legs, particularly if I have any injury. That's me!

*Move, right arm and hand, Move!*

The occupational therapist team set out to create some arm and hand functionality. Retraining arms and hands is significantly more difficult than working with legs because the upper body has many more nerves. My right shoulder was frozen. In therapy, we did repetitive exercises and played children's board games (such as Connect Four), with me trying to use my right hand.

Writing was at the top of the occupational therapists' to do list. Remember when you or your children were three or four years old and learning to write on wide-lined paper? That was me. But my right hand just wasn't functioning properly so I was getting nowhere. It was frustrating. Furthermore, using the right arm continued to be painful due to my frozen shoulder.

*But wait – could we try left-handed?*

I started to think about my youth. I could play ping pong with my left hand, not as well as my right, but I could play. And when playing singles tennis as a righty, I would shift the tennis racquet on the run to my left hand to reach backhand shots I would otherwise have missed. That triggered an idea.

One day I let the therapists know that I wanted to try to learn to write lefty. Though the therapists resisted, I was determined to try.

(A speech pathologist more recently told me therapists should have encouraged me to try my left hand immediately. They also should have encouraged me to turn pages in a book the opposite way.)

Perhaps the therapists hadn't given up on my right hand just yet.

*Becoming a lefty was working!*

Everyone but me was surprised. The therapists were puzzled, as are many people to this day when they hear that I just changed hands. All of a sudden, I was a lefty! *Now I am getting someplace!*

*You never know what's before you. And I never would have thought that my childhood ping pong games would provide a way back!*

My biggest left-handed writing issues were trying to write a check mark, an S or a Z. I would write them backwards. Now I do it as a joke—to remind myself of where I was.

△

*It's party time!*

On Saturday nights, in an effort to increase my verbal skills and to jump start our non-existent social life, Debbie started to invite family and friends to parties in my room. Since I had a private room, the nursing home gave Debbie permission to bring wine to enhance the party atmosphere.

In retrospect, I think the parties helped caregiver Debbie cope with the entire situation, created a little normalcy, and gave her a bit of a social life. It gave her something to look forward to. Debbie liked to party. Why not? She deserved it.

The evenings usually ended early for me. When our guests arrived, I was sitting up and chatting a bit, but I always felt at a loss for words.

I had very little to say. Today, when I visit someone in the hospital or a retirement facility I still feel the same way. I guess I don't have a good bedside manner as a patient or a visitor.

Though I wasn't allowed to drink the vino, I appreciated the food which was always great. Debbie brought in food from some of our favorite restaurants. Invariably, I fell asleep soon after eating as the parties rolled on. And after several weeks of daily speech therapy, often twice a day, my speaking ability was making strides.

*The big push was to return life to reasonable normalcy as soon as possible.*

This would be important for any caregiver in our situation – stabilize and create a modicum of normalcy!

*It's early, but I am clearly on the way back. Halleluiah!*

# CHAPTER 6
# THE SUN BEGINS TO SHINE

*I was progressing.*

The facial drooping I had initially experienced was improving and my face looked more normal, so Debbie told me. I still hadn't seen myself! At the nursing home, mirrors were off limits and since I was not independently mobile, I had no way to look at myself. Frankly, I didn't even think to look. (Pretty out of it, wouldn't you say?) Wondering about shaving? I was using an electric razor, sitting down, with a nurse's assistance.

I do remember realizing that my towel drooling had largely stopped since I no longer had a permanent towel for a bib. The aides made a big deal about its removal. You'd have to be blind not to notice!

*Still, a nursing home!*

Other than the nursing home staff and the therapists treating me, I didn't speak with anyone except my visitors, who were quite numerous. Since Stamford was so central to Debbie's world, her son Keith, her three brothers, and of course, her mother Ruthie and father Bucky would pop in. (Debbie's father also was in a wheelchair since losing his legs to diabetes a few years earlier. Actually, his legs had been amputated a few days before the Easter Sunday I met him). Many friends also came by.

The Mediplex staff encouraged me to develop friends in the facility—after all; I would be there for a few months. The staff also wanted me to eat in the dining room but I would have none of it. The residents in rooms near mine seemed so old and in many cases, feeble.

*I stayed in my little private world. Call it hiding!*

There was an exception, I thought. I had noticed a gentleman about my age, a professional - looking type in the rehab gym room. One day I asked an aide to wheel me up to him so we might meet. As I started to speak, he shocked me by angrily waving me away! I was taken aback and disappointed. So much for my try at friendship at the nursing home!

Later, a nurse told me that the gentleman had indeed suffered a stroke but that he had permanently lost his ability to speak and was getting violent. A few weeks later, I heard that his business had to be sold and that his family was forced to institutionalize him.

*By God, that could have been me!*

*

When I first arrived at the nursing home, I was incapable of doing anything for myself. Aides would dress and undress me. Since I was incontinent, they accompanied me to the bathroom. It all was bad. For several weeks, I wore a diaper at night until after a time I noticed that it was consistently dry. That's when the aides eliminated the diaper and opted for an extra rubber bed pad.

*Bathing in the nursing home - I'm not getting bathed every day – far from it – UGH!*

I was only being bathed twice a week. It was unacceptable, but not so rare in nursing homes, as I later learned. Always proactive, Debbie had words with the administrator. She managed to get the schedule adjusted to bathing every other day. Not enough, but a step in the right direction and, the best she could do.

On bathing days, an aide pushed my wheelchair into a big shower room and transferred me to a wheelchair designed for the shower. It had a frame with openings so water could drain. Then the aide positioned me under a large shower head to shower me. The aide undressed me down to my shorts before turning the water on and rinsing, soaping and rinsing me again while I sat in the chair. It reminded me of a clothes washer! Toward the end of the shower, the attendants had me remove my shorts and I cleaned my genital area before being wrapped up in a towel like a mummy. After that, they took me back to my room and dressed me. I was happy to feel cleaner.

Though there was nothing unseemly, I felt almost abused by this process. The experience varied by aide so I requested certain aides by name, sometimes to no avail. Thinking back, I had mixed feelings about having more showers: I didn't really look forward to shower day, even though I wanted to bathe.

*A small victory but neither Debbie nor I were happy.*

*

Soon after arriving at the nursing home, a shoe salesperson arrived in my room to take measurements for sneakers that closed with Velcro. After listening to the salesperson, I angrily dismissed him.

"No, I will not wear these even if I have to go barefoot," I told him in halting speech. My stubbornness was showing. To me, those shoes represented the ultimate cave-in to my condition. The nursing home aides were not happy with me.

*Tough shit! There's no way I'm wearing those shoes.*

So I set out to learn to tie my shoelaces. This was not an easy task with a barely functioning right hand. Spending hours trying to relearn, at times the aides watched me struggle, and ultimately tied my laces, so I could get down to the rehab room. Other times when I was not scheduled they let me struggle. When I tied my laces it was hard because I had to lean forward to stretch my arms to tie my laces, which then affected my balance, even in a sitting position.

You wouldn't think it but tying laces is dependent on many subtle factors: my angle when sitting, how low I was sitting, whether the chair had arms and so on. Even today, depending on the chair that I am sitting in, I can have difficulty tying my laces, particularly as the laces stretch from wear and I have to double tie them.

*But I refuse to wear Velcro shoes!*

\*

Meanwhile, I was making progress on the stairs. It must have been a month of practice before I began to feel more comfortable. For my safety, a therapist and an aide worked with me. I would climb seven stairs to a landing, then rest before coming back down. Eventually, I would climb to a second level, in total the equivalent of a full flight. Of course, I held onto the sturdy banisters and the therapy team guided me up and down, holding me with a harness.

\*

After about six weeks at Mediplex, the administrator said I could have a pass to leave for a few hours. Debbie was happy that we could start to do something on weekends. The night before my first pass I panicked.

*The SUV's too high!*

How was I going to climb into Debbie's big Jeep Grand Cherokee SUV? Sitting in a wheelchair, I imagined that I would not be able to get into the vehicle. *Was I screwed up!*

*It looked sooo far up. I can't do that! Funny how incorrect perceptions can affect you!*

I was so panicked that I called her to say she shouldn't come to the nursing home if she planned to take me out. I didn't want a big argument.

*I was clearly in a panic!*

The staff assured me that one of the therapists would give me a hand. They did! Once I was standing upright, I was able to get in with assistance. With the aide, it wasn't that hard at all!

Even so, I was afraid during our first few car trips around Stamford and New Canaan. I didn't want to get out of the car. Though we did have a wheelchair in the boot, I wasn't interested in getting out.

*What if Debbie couldn't get me back in?*

But that was resolved after a few extra practice sessions. The aides stopped assisting us, rather just watched and I was able to get into and out of the SUV.

Soon Mediplex extended the passes so we could go out to lunch. That experience helped me to understand just how restricted life would be if I was confined to a wheelchair, particularly in the Northeast where the terrain is hilly and many older buildings lack good handicap access.

As we tried to go to our favorite restaurants, we saw things I had never noticed before as a healthy person. Narrow hallways and doors, stairs without banisters, and tables placed too close to navigate a wheelchair were typical examples. One restaurant we had frequented often had only one little table near the door where we could sit. In that place all of the other tables were up at least several steps without a banister. Before the stroke, I never gave it a second thought. Navigating a wheel chair on some of the hilly streets of Connecticut also was an issue. Fortunately, Debbie was (and is) superbly fit.

*Something to Do, an Outing*

As a weekend afternoon activity, we started to visit the lovely sculpture garden and park at the Pepsi Co corporate headquarters in Purchase, N.Y., just over the Connecticut state border. In this angelic setting, employees sat outside at lunch in nice weather. On weekends, when the buildings are officially closed, the public uses the grounds as a park. There, too, the parkland is set on a slope leading down to a picturesque pond surrounded by manicured woodlands. Debbie wheeled me around, sometimes jogging as she did.

By early spring, I could celebrate other signs of progress. My speech was more normal and becoming more natural. (I still had difficulty repeating five or six word lists—a problem that continues to this day, but I work around it by writing lists).

And back at the nursing home, I was improving my ability to walk with a quad cane. My left-handed writing ability continued to improve and, thank God, my internal plumbing was now working better.

*In April, the sun began to shine!*

# CHAPTER 7
# EMOTIONS AND COPING

About two months into my three-month stay, the nursing home began giving me Saturday night passes to go home. The administrator explained that I needed to begin the process of readjusting to our home as my stay was quickly coming to an end.

Frankly, I wasn't real happy about the thought of going home, having become quite comfortable with my surroundings, the attention I was getting in therapy and the sheltered life I led.

*Funny how your psyche changes! When I got there and realized I was in a nursing home, I was anxious to leave. Now I wanted to stay!*

I was concerned that my progress at home would stop or at least slow significantly. Additionally, during the week, I would be alone all day since Debbie was teaching. And like many people, mostly men, being alone is not my favorite state. Outpatient rehabilitation was yet to be organized and driving was out. I would be stuck.

*Is this what "house arrest" feels like?*

Fortunately we were able to get the nursing home to extend my stay a few weeks more than they had originally planned to give me additional time for therapy. Still being very sick and needy, I was comfortable staying put.

Thinking back, the fact that I felt so insecure that I wanted to stay in a nursing home longer seems unbelievable.

*Was that me? Na - that must have been somebody else!*

**A Big Coping Strategy**

Though my therapists had been helping me relearn to walk stairs, I always had a banister. I had not been successful without a banister. My balance was still way off. However, at home we only had one banister on the lower level staircase, which led up to the main living level though we did have two on the stairs up to the master bedroom on the upper level. So, at a minimum, I would have to go up or down at least one flight to enter or leave the condo. Certainly we could have installed another banister to make it easier. That was particularly true since the wall that did not have a banister was straight. But we didn't.

Fortunately the banister was on the left side so going up was no issue with my handicap. I could hold the banister for support – and at the beginning I held it onto it "for dear life." Of course, that left me with a big problem - getting back down.

I wanted to learn to cope. If a solution wasn't found it would have made me forever dependent on dual banisters for egress. There are a heck of a lot of situations with only one banister, particularly in older buildings and homes. Even worse, there are staircases with no banisters. But that's another story. So learning to cope with a single banister was important to living an independent life.

*There was only one answer - go down backwards!*

Preparing for my first Saturday night pass, I was able to get the therapists to assist with my initial efforts at backwards stair walking. As usual they held me with a harness as I descended. But here again, there is a lesson to be learned.

It is one thing to do a task like this under the supervision of a trained therapist with a harness for support and quite another doing it at home with no therapist and no harness, particularly for the first time. When the therapist was there I felt secure, when she wasn't I was nervous.

The first time I peered down from the main level of our condo to the entry below it was visually nerve-racking. Amazing, I had never given it a second thought.

*Damn, this is steep! I never thought that when I was healthy.*

To make it worse, the stairs at Mediplex had landings in the middle of each flight so as one looked down you were only looking at seven steps. At home, however I was looking down an entire flight. *Scary stuff!*

In the beginning, I tightly held the single banister, walking down backwards one-step-at-a-time, bringing both feet to each stair before venturing again. And Debbie was in front of me on a lower stair at the beginning. However, as time went by, I became more comfortable with the stairs and I started to develop a rhythm where I could just go down as if I was walking forwards.

*It worked!!*

**But a cautionary note - in a new location, I still revert to the one-step-at-a-time process to avoid falling. Once I am more comfortable with a particular set of stairs, my rhythm gradually kicks in. It's actually not that hard when you get the knack of it.**

**But please, please - should you try this, be very careful!**

Invariably, when I walk backwards in a public location there are stares of wonderment. While I can't imagine that I'm the first person to walk down backwards most people apparently haven't witnessed it.

A funny anecdote occurred a few years ago while visiting the Vatican in Rome. Debbie and I had taken our friend, Father John's, suggestion to visit the remarkable but not well known Scavi, which is the area beneath the Vatican. Some of the most famous Popes in history are buried there among the secret caverns. Absolutely fascinating!

To reach the underground Scavi, one has to descend a very steep and narrow concrete staircase, and you guessed it, there was only one banister. When I looked down this foreboding entrance I thought to myself, "can and should I do this? If this is what the beginning is, what's it going to be like once we get inside?"

*I don't want to miss this experience! Screw it, I'll do it. I can always bale if it gets too hairy.*

I descended first, and the eyes of several members of our group seemed to nearly pop as I made my way down backwards. A few clapped as I reached the bottom. We quickly bonded and the strangers were friendlier and made way for me as we made our way through the narrow corridors to peek into the darkened and spooky chambers. Navigating some of the winding and narrow passageways under the Vatican was equally challenging, but so worth it. But I'll admit to taking a deep breath when it was over! I had done it and not skipped anything. *Stroke Victor!*

Just as an aside, so you are aware, to visit the Scavi takes planning. One has to make reservations well in advance as the availability is very limited. Because of the narrow walk ways, tours are limited to about twelve people. So it's sure a lot different than going through the Vatican with your closest 25,000 friends. We did both since they are different experiences. So should you, but I would suggest doing the tours on different days if you have the time.

*Back at the ranch*

During my first weekend at home you would probably think that it must have been wonderful. **Not true!** It felt both weird and off-putting, like I was a visitor to our home. There were no therapists with harnesses and I was shakily using my quad cane and a wheel chair that Debbie had rented.

You can see why the nursing home was prudent to start giving Saturday night adjustment passes. Kudos to them!

*Those first few weeks, when I returned to the nursing home on Sunday night, I was glad to be back. I was safe! They were taking care of me.*

Looking back, I had changed, at least for the time being. Wow!

# CHAPTER 8
# HOME ALONE — IS THIS MY DEAL? - *YIKES!*

The day was here and now, I had run out of stall tactics.

*Hard to believe, but the day had finally come!*

And I wasn't the least bit happy! My bags were packed and Debbie made her final trip to Mediplex. I was insecure and nervous about what the future held. Debbie would be teaching and I'd be in our condo alone.

Before moving back she had arranged for the Visiting Nurses (VNA) to start coming the house while she lined up bona fide outpatient therapy. There wasn't much in Ridgefield. However, she had found Main Street Rehabilitation in Danbury for the out-patient services which turned out to be brilliant. The facility had a wonderful local reputation.

It was well equipped and staffed – that was the good news. The bad news - they had no openings, so I had been placed on a waiting list.

*So I was cooling my heels at home and feeling lost!*

The VNA visited our home two or three times per week, each time for somewhere between 30 and 45 minutes. They were an earnest bunch of woman but there wasn't very much they could do in our house. They stretched my shoulder, arm, and leg, took my blood pressure and taught me a few exercises but, as a practical matter, they kept me company. I must confess, I welcomed the visits; **I felt lost at home.** It was such a contrast to the constant activity of the nursing home with all of its therapy sessions, and family and friends who would daily visit.

Debbie had set up a wonderful office for me in our family room on the main level and though I was starting to work again, I was home alone. I never really liked that very much! It's interesting, today so many people work out of their homes including my daughter, Amy, and son-in-law, Pete, but I don't know how they do it. It's not for me. I don't like the isolation, and it's too easy to get distracted by non-business stuff.

We were constantly on the phone with Main Street to see when they would be able to squeeze me into their therapy rotation. What made it difficult was that we wanted neurologically trained therapists with stroke experience. And they don't come a dime a dozen!

*It was important to get therapists who had the correct training and skill sets for my issues, which is another lesson to be noted.* Neurological problems are best dealt with by someone who has been trained with that orientation. Debbie's idea!

Main Street had therapists who met our criteria but they were initially booked. It took nearly a month to get my initial screening appointments with the appropriate therapists – but Carrie and Kathy who had neurological experience finally became available.

Next step was to focus on transportation since Debbie wasn't there and I wasn't driving. Ridgefield being somewhat rural had very limited taxi service, which was prohibitively expensive. Anyway, no taxi driver seemed interested in our fifteen-mile local business, preferring the more lucrative airport runs. Desperate, we ran an advertisement for a driver in the local weekly newspaper, *The Ridgefield Press.*

God was watching! A woman answered the advertisement, and she herself was going to Main Street Rehab for a serious hand ailment. She was a most giving soul and we made a financial arrangement with her. Remarkably, she even agreed to take me on those days when she had none of her own treatments, as she wasn't working at the time. We certainly appreciated her assistance.

My initial schedule consisted of daily physical and occupational therapy, aqua therapy three times a week in a heated pool, and some limited speech and psychological therapy. It was a chock full schedule.

*After a stroke, water therapy in a warm pool is a fantastic activity.* I was able to walk in the pool unaided and also without the assistance of a cane. The water's buoyancy was my protection from falls. The therapists gave me exercises to do in the pool and free time to just walk around.

*Triumphantly, I walked around feeling independent – I never wanted it to end, loving the independence that the pool afforded me. This was a game-changer!*

And with this growing feeling of confidence, I made some excellent strides both walking and also with my stair egress. The only downside was the considerable time it took to change clothes for the pool sessions. However, since there were other patients in the open area of the locker room a bit of camaraderie soon developed.

I was uncomfortable with the psychological therapy and didn't want to dwell on the situation as it was.

*I wasn't looking back. How do you undo something like a stroke? It's history, move on!*

In retrospect, without planning it, my modus operandi was just to move forward one-day-at a time in a self-directed way. I have always believed that by not delving into psychological issues, I prevented myself from getting depressed, which was critically important to the recovery. Psychological sessions disturbed me, and certainly at that fragile stage, I thought it best to pass. Psychologists would probably disagree, and maybe they would be correct. This is me.

Sessions in the well-equipped gym took the place of other therapy as I was slowly improving. The gym was staffed by an excellent exercise physiologist team, and I started going there nearly every day. Going to the gym was enjoyable due to the friendliness of the staff and patients and of course, it helped me. I spent time on the

## Part III

# *Points of Transformation*

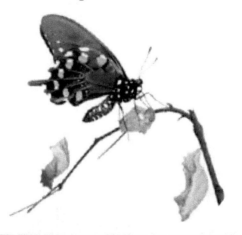

When you find your self cocooned
in
isolation
and cannot find your way
out of the darkness,
remember
that this is similar to the place
where
caterpillars go to grow their wings.

*Unknown*

# CHAPTER 9

## DRIVING AT NASCAR, NO – THE HILLS OF SAN FRANCISCO, YES

When I was handicapped in Ridgefield there was nowhere to go without a car. I couldn't even get down our driveway to walk on the street because our townhouse was built on a hill, so the driveway reflected that topography.

Yes, when I had been healthy we often walked to town from where we lived, but I didn't have a prayer of doing it alone. There were several steep hills and a few rough patches.

*No independence.*

Something had to be done about this situation! Driving was the answer.

Before entertaining the thought of driving, I needed a driver evaluation to assess my eyesight and reflexes. Once again, Main Street in Danbury had the answer. They had this giant driver evaluation machine which tested your sight, your peripheral vision, and also your reaction times for safety.

I had marveled at this giant contraption for months, whenever I walked around it, though rarely had I seen anybody using it. I kept wondering what it would be like to be tested. And more importantly, would I pass?

*Would I ever be able to drive again?*

If not, it would be a disastrous problem in rural Ridgefield! We certainly would have to move. However, I am not sure where we would go since there were very few places, if any, in Fairfield

County, Connecticut, where I could get along without a car when it was combined with challenged walking.

Testing day came and I was nervous! I sat in the machine and was shown various light patterns to see if I reacted fast enough to the stimuli, assuming I saw them at all. I was tested with and without glasses in order to get a full picture of my abilities. As the lights blinked, I saw some patterns, but missed quite a lot of others. On other occasions, I saw the lights but by the time I reacted they were gone. I was so nervous that the test had to be redone with my glasses on; actually I probably failed the first time so they gave me a second chance. Fair enough! Ultimately, I passed, but the tests indicated a loss of right side peripheral vision that was, fortunately, correctible with a new eyeglass prescription.

*Now here's a lesson.* **When I walked around, I was unaware of my sight losses.** *I didn't realize that my sight had diminished on my right side so having the driver evaluation was really important. But now, with my new glasses,* I was ready to go.

Here is my one-step-at-a-time solution for driving, the process I worked out. And thinking about it -- if you were teaching your children or grandchildren to drive, this might be a prudent approach to adapt also.

I asked myself under what circumstances I would drive. Before the stroke, I drove in rural and suburban areas with and without traffic. Since I was from New York and comfortable driving there, I also drove in New York at peak and off-peak hours and in unfamiliar locations when we traveled. So, I would be driving in several environments, but initially just locally around the greater Ridgefield area. So, to fully recover my skills might take as many as five or six phases.

Let's start in Ridgefield, our home and a town whose Main Street looks like it is right out of a modern day Currier and Ives, part suburban and part rural. So, it was on these un-crowded roads that I began to retrain myself as a driver. In Phase One, I started driving during daylight non-rush hour times. Town speed limits were in the 35 mile-an-hour range and I was very cautious.

*That's all I would have needed – to be pulled over by the police.*

On my first outing, I was very cautious backing our Plymouth Acclaim sedan out of the garage. I drove for about fifteen minutes. I wanted to get a feel of the car again, so I just drove around the area and came home feeling happy.

*Guess what, no crash! I could still drive. Yippy!*

Over the next several weeks, I increased the time I drove. I often drove on Route 35, a winding two-lane road heading towards horse country in North and South Salem, New York. I was practicing daily after being dropped off by my driver to increase my comfort level. I also started to practice my parallel parking. Growing up in New York where parking spaces are at a premium, I had learned to "park on a dime." But now with a still stiff neck, this wasn't so easy. I spent some time practicing in remote areas of parking lots to get my distance perception reoriented. It worked. At this point, Debbie didn't know about my little "joy rides" since she would have freaked! Thinking back, I was like a kid who steals the family car.

It was time to graduate to Phase Two, which was driving in the dark, but still not in rush hour. The month was late November and it gets dark in Ridgefield at about 4:30 p.m. I tested my skills, nighttime driving eyesight, and ability driving on roads which would not have lots of traffic. The new glasses were doing their job!

I felt confident about my driving, so I brought Debbie in on my little driving secret, and she immediately accompanied me on a successful run. After a few weeks and with a higher comfort level, it was time for Phase Three, which was to drive during daylight rush-hour. That said, Ridgefield is not New York, so there wasn't much serious traffic. Eventually, I graduated into evening rush hour feeling more secure, Phase Four.

Now, driving regularly and increasing my independence, I was going to Main Street under my own steam. Some of the therapy had ceased and though spending time with the exercise physiologist, I was returning home earlier in the afternoon. This allowed me to work more hours in the telemarketing business. I was screening sales people, among other things.

A few weeks later, Andy, my business partner and I had a business trip to San Francisco to raise venture capital where I had to rent an SUV and drive the hills around and in San Francisco. Debbie had taken a medical leave for six months to catch her breath and had come along.

A business trip, even accompanied, and driving in a challenging urban location, was Phase Five. We arrived late at night in San Francisco Airport and the place was mobbed, though I don't know why. Just San Fran!

When we got to the car rental counter, the only vehicle that was available was a large SUV, which we really didn't want or need. They told me I could have it, or to get in line. And since there were no cars this looked like a long wait. Actually, the only reason they offered us that vehicle ahead of the other renters was that I was an elite member of the National Rental Car loyalty program – Emerald Club. That transaction got quite a few nasty stares but there's a reason to be an elite member in an auto rental program or an airline program, for that matter. We were lucky that my elite status had not yet been cancelled due to non-use.

I can't remember why Debbie didn't drive; it certainly would have made perfect sense in unfamiliar territory with a huge vehicle, but she didn't. And Andy also, when he arrived!

*I was probably so stubborn and fixated on recovery that no one wanted to get in my way!*

After driving a few of the wicked hills of San Francisco, I announced that my comfort level was at pre - stroke levels. The last phase had been achieved! When I think about it today, I probably wasn't all that good a driver then, but I wasn't all that bad either.

*Heck, we made it back to the airport with the rented SUV in one piece!*

# CHAPTER 10
# SOME OF MY MOST IMPORTANT LESSONS

**CONTRAST THESE:**

*"I am going to walk down the nursing home hallway today." Stumbling, "I can't do it. Damn! I can only take a step. Help, I need help, Shit. I can't even walk those few steps! How will I get down the hall?"*

**Outcome** - I feel dejected, depressed, frustrated and unhappy, **a failure**. I can't do it!

*VS*

*"I am going to take **one step today.** I do. There, I did it. **Success!"***

**Outcome** - I am smiling and satisfied. I accomplished my objective. Let's try for two tomorrow. I'm in a good mood.

⌂

Picture it. Here I was – sick as heck! When I had the stroke, I figured I would be back to new in a year. That seemed forever and so that seemed reasonable. There were all those months, all those weeks and all of those days to recover.

But you know something - it wasn't even close! Not by a country mile.

*But what did I know - I never had a stroke before!! And actually I didn't know anyone else who had one either.*

How I reconciled this with keeping my spirits up begins with the first and most important lesson that I learned!

*And if you take away only one lesson from this book – **take away this one.***

**GO ONE-STEP-AT-A-TIME! And think it through, you or your caregiver.**

Recently, I heard an injured veteran of the war in Afghanistan who was being interviewed on TV say the same thing – go one-step-at-a-time - and I felt good for him. Don't misunderstand – I felt really bad that what happened to him, happened, but I felt good that he had it right. He would succeed as long as he held to the mantra and didn't get impatient or frustrated!

So what does this exactly mean when you are where I was after a massive stroke or any other major disability? Simply, it meant:

I take one step at physical therapy, for example, and I am satisfied and I have a smile on my face – I just won the four minute mile – there are cheers and accolades – can't you hear them!

Tomorrow, I take two steps – and I'm happy, and I won a second four minute mile race. I am all smiles – more accolades. Well, the next day, maybe, I repeat the two - step objective, and I am still happy, with a smile, because maybe I did two better steps than the day before. Or maybe, I had a not so good day – don't fret – move forward.

The next day, I walk three steps, and I am happy and so on; and the fifth day – maybe I repeat the three - step objective.

Now look, on the weekend – the sixth and seventh day – I didn't have therapy, so no progress was made but I need my rest. More importantly, my injured brain needed the rest to heal. There is research to support that.

Now comes Monday, *"I have to get hustling again!"*

Monday, maybe I regress a little – it's harder to smile but I don't give up – stay with me! But, but, but – that next day I have to focus just a bit more and not get grumpy or discouraged. Keep going!

*Focus and do your thing! And this can go on for some time, just keep moving forward ...*

*"With a smile in your heart!"*

Just think of a stock rally on Wall Street. Even in the most bullish of times – there are down days! You just want to be sure that you are having more up days than down days.

**The key is to keep having small wins, even tiny wins, but at all cost, avoid the big depressing failure**s which lead to depression! Keep smiling on the down days, taking it with a grain of salt. (Just not too big of a grain, because we should be on a low-salt diet after a stroke!)

Now, I am sure that this all seems painfully slow and maybe simplistic. You're absolutely right, but it's darn important. I had to accept it, but in reality it's pretty tough. So don't be surprised.

**It's not so easy to keep smiling when it's going slowly or barely going at all.**

*I got frustrated just like everyone else. But fortunately I didn't let it get the better of me!*

It was slow, it was very slow sometimes. Painfully slow. With faith and hard work, I mean hard, I prevailed. Why can't you?

**Quantity and Quality**

Let's talk about another dimension of one step-at-a-time recovery dynamics -- quantity and quality.

Of course, you have heard those terms before, perhaps in reference to other more pleasant things. In this instance – what does it mean and how did I meaningfully implement it?

First of all, I created a baseline, a starting point. For me and many other stroke survivors in a wheelchair, I was not standing at all. So, first I had to be able to stand. Could I stand straight or was I swaying. Could I accomplish standing without support, or did I have to hold on?

Standing straight is quality, swaying is not; hanging on for support is not. One-step-at-a-time, I want to stand straight without support.

Then I took a step with a quad cane for support but it was halting. That's quantity, not quality. I accomplished it, which is great, but it wasn't such a good step. It was halting, and not a normal step. It needs to be improved. That's quantity, not quality! The quality has to go up.

Next, I take two steps; the first is improved but the second is shaky. Again, quantity, not quality, but improving quality because the first step was better. Or, in taking the step, did I raise my affected foot too high, which is a typical post - stroke thing. Or do I land on my ankle, so that my weak ankle twists?

Of course, more positively, is it a normal length step or a baby step? Sometimes two baby steps are better than one longer single step particularly if that step is what I call "sloppy" or awkward!

Or, when I take two steps, is the second step as long as the first step? Or can I take the first step without some kind of physical support, but as I bring the second foot forward, did I have to grab for support? Early on, I remember feeling as though I was going to fall if I didn't grab for support quickly.

Eventually, I got down the parallel bars under my own steam, and then the hall, and then I walked the floor. But, it was all done, one-step-at-a-time, <u>and slowly</u>.

*I'm thinking, get some quantity but not at the complete expense of quality. Quantity has to come first. Quality comes second. You have to take the step before it can be judged.*

*And eventually I got my quality up, walking more naturally though still with a cane in those early days.*

I hope this is clear since it is a bit complicated. What's the movie that Meryl Streep and Alec Baldwin were in a few years ago? *"It's Complicated"* In their case, what was complicated were the dynamics of a later-in–life-marriage. In my case it was getting off my rump!

For walking or any other task there are lots of factors which are intermixed as I sorted out quantity and quality. Well, it was indeed complicated, but not insurmountable.

*If I can do it, you can do it!*

Going one-step-at-a-time and thinking about quantity and quality, I worked hard keeping that smile on my face, which leads to another important lesson.

## Mr. Grinch, Get Lost!

It sounds simple to a healthy person, probably because they luckily haven't had to think about it. But disposing of Mr. Grinch is really tough. And the more serious the disability, the tougher it can be. But sooo what – smile!  As I did or tried to.

Because if I don't, I risk becoming Mr. Grinch!

*There are some darn good reasons to smile, even if I don't think so.*

*First of all – I feel better when I smile than when I am Mr. Grinch!*

I am sure that there are psychological studies that say I am healthier and my body feels better, when I smile. So my body should heal faster. It certainly will not heal more slowly.

But secondly, and here is the really important next reason to smile and project a good mood:

*I found that my therapists worked harder with me if I was in a good mood.*

Put yourself in the therapist's shoes. Here are two situations:

We are in the rehab gym. Mr. Bob is ready to go, even practicing on his own with a smile on his face. He is happy and joking, but over there in the corner,

There is Mr. Grinch, with a long face! He is going through the motions or even worse, maybe he's just sitting there, just plain pissed off or depressed!

Now, of course, the professional therapist is going to give both their allotted time, but who do you think is going to have a better outcome! Who might actually make some progress today? And who do you think the therapist would rather be working with?

*I'll put my money on the smiling, happy, Mr. Bob patient every time.*

**I WANTED THAT PERSON TO BE ME** – sooo you want that to be you!

# CHAPTER 11

# SMALL LESSONS THAT MAKE A BIG DIFFERENCE

When I was healthy, there were a lot of things that I just took for granted and didn't give a second thought. We all do. Some are pretty mundane, but with a disability, it's a whole different ballgame. You have to think about this and that, and then create solutions. Let me describe a few:

## NAILS

Since my right hand wasn't working properly, I couldn't hold a nail clipper or scissors safely. So, I wasn't able to cut my nails. A fix was needed!

If your partner can cut your nails, great! But if you are like me and your spouse has always gotten manicures and pedicures, and is a disaster at cutting nails -- think bloody fingers, then its manicure and pedicure time!

I, like many men, am self-conscious at a nail salon. Nineteen years ago, I would be the only male there. It's changed somewhat in more recent years but we are still in the great minority. It turns out to be a nice small luxury. I felt clean and comfortable, but I was still glad when it was over. On weekends, getting our nails done became a joint activity. Still, I was self-conscious, as nice as the people were.

The interesting thing is the number of women who compliment me for having my nails done. They often would, and today still do, say things like, *"I wish my boyfriend or husband did that. You look so clean."* There's a lesson, guys!

Besides nail maintenance, I had an issue with soft, breaking and splitting nails. One or several of my blood pressure medications was causing that. The fix, nail hardeners and high doses of Biotin suggested by a hand surgeon to strengthen the nails! Today, I take 5 mgs of Biotin twice a day.

## TEETH

After my stroke, I was having trouble vigorously brushing my teeth and as a result, was developing periodontal disease, which is an inflammation of the tooth supporting structures. My gums were bleeding excessively, so it wasn't a good situation. There started to be a risk of losing some teeth.

The fix, first, we found a periodontal dental practice and I started going for quarterly cleanings. Second, I started exclusively using prescription or professional grade fluoride toothpaste and requested the periodontist to give me a prescription.

Just as a note, there is non-prescription high fluoride toothpaste available, Control X, in some dental offices. That works, but is very expensive for toothpaste. There is also a prescription grade generic, gotten with a dentist's prescription. Both have worked for me. These specialized toothpastes are worth the extra cost and insurance may cover the prescription item. Think about it: people of all ages do not get much fluoride today, if they drink bottled water. This solves it.

And third, I started flossing my teeth. With one hand challenged, I found Flossers, which are one-handed tooth flossing plastic gadgets. They are probably not as good as traditional flossing, but a lot better than nothing.

## ESCALATORS

It was the late 90's and I was starting to travel on business again. I was visiting the home office of our company, Interactive Teleservices in Lincoln, Nebraska. Our office had moved from its original home in the basement of a building near the Capital in Lincoln to the Gold's building, which was nearer to the University of Nebraska campus. The building is a beautifully designed department store that went south, so the real estate had been redeveloped into offices. We were on the fifth floor and ordinarily we took either an elevator or escalator to get upstairs. Because we ran two shifts we typically worked long and late hours.

I had gone out for a drink with a friend who wasn't in the company not realizing that the elevators stopped running at 5 p.m. Upon my return, I did not know how to navigate an escalator and was alone. With no one around, I became very perturbed. No one knew that I had a predicament because this was the pre-cell phone era. I had to get into the building to get my luggage and finish a few things. Still on a cane, I'm in the empty lobby with no elevator and only the escalator available!

*How do I do this with only one useful hand holding a cane, and the escalator rapidly moving?*

After looking at the escalator for a few minutes, I decided to throw the cane on the escalator and then use my hand to grab the moving rail to stabilize myself. In this case, I always lead with my good foot to attain the best stability. Even doing that, I nearly fell getting on the escalator and again as I got off. Since I had to get up to the fifth floor I wound up doing the same thing several times, improving as I repeated it. I did it. Quite shaken, I got back to the office safely.

*You just have to do what you have to do!*

One of my business partners helped out as I left for the evening, taking my luggage out. Now I can use an escalator easily but I still haven't learned how to handle the luggage on the escalator. It's on my to – do list, since elevators are sometimes not conveniently located, particularly in airports.

## HOTELS WITH SHOWERS ABOVE THE BATHTUB

A few years ago we went to a beautiful inn/hotel - Keswick Hall in the horse, fox hound and wine country of Virginia. It was located about a 15 minute drive on back roads from Thomas Jefferson's home, Monticello. It had been a long day, starting in Hanover, MD, a bedroom community half way between Washington D.C. and Baltimore. We had exercised in Annapolis, and then confirmed arrangements for a business meeting in Williamsburg, VA., about three to four hours away. Then we were to go to Keswick Hall.

Arriving at the hotel near 8 p.m., after going thru Richmond, Virginia rush-hour traffic, we checked in and went to dinner. There were no rooms with stand-alone showers available for that evening. When we returned to the room a few hours later, I realized just how difficult the situation was. The tub walls were very high and encased in a wooden frame. Quaint as it was, it was super inconvenient. We decided to deal with it, though it was extraordinarily awkward.

After several unsuccessful and awkward attempts, I sat on the tub frame and balanced while Debbie tightly held my one side. I grabbed a bar that was attached to the wall and pulled my first leg into the tub. Debbie then grabbed the other leg that was still out of the tub and shoved it into the tub. *Yikes!*

If Debbie had lost her footing or something I would have fallen and probably injured myself. Getting out was a bit easier but essentially a reverse of the first process. In the morning, after repeating this process I went down to change rooms. The staff was quite accommodating after I explained my situation. First they suggested an adapted room but I explained that we just needed a room with a separate shower, which they sorted out as some other guests had checked out. We were very appreciative!

When I have these situations, I often meet the nicest people like Bill. He moved us, and so we had a chance to chat. He told me that he had retired from the Pentagon where he was an engineer and was now working to put his last child through college. He acknowledged that the high frames and elegant tubs had resulted in other people slipping on the damp floors if they were not careful. He also told me about his family history of heart/stroke problems so I told him about the future development of my stroke recovery site and he was real excited.

I said – stand by!

Today, we also stay in many normal hotels where there are traditional bath/shower designs. In these hotels I reach up and use the shower curtain rod to assist in getting into and out of the tub. However, before using the rod I look to be sure that it is securely fastened to the wall. On occasion, I find that the rod is flimsily attached, is secured by a spring type mechanism or the screws are loose or missing. The rod is then not safe to utilize.

When the bar is not an option I look for something else to hold as I enter and leave the bathtub with the shower. Each location requires some accommodations; I just look at the situation and make my adjustments.

After enough of these experiences, I now take more care to request a room with a shower instead of the combo if they are available. Also, we request a non-skid shower mat to prevent slipping.

## ATTENDING A CONVENTION IN ATLANTA

A few years ago I attended the National Association of Gifted Children national convention in Atlanta. I have a rule when attending conventions since I became disabled: **always stay at the convention headquarters hotel,** even if it's more expensive. This significantly increases convenience.

There always is more than enough walking and usually, schlepping of books and marketing materials. In this case the sessions that I attended were at the hotel but the exposition was at the convention center in a different part of Atlanta - a complication.

Atlanta was madness the evening of the convention opening. Two professional teams – the Falcons and the Atlanta Hawks were scheduled. Traffic was at a standstill and many people were on the streets walking. To make it more interesting, there was road construction in the downtown area.

As we were to leave late in the afternoon, I realized that to get to the bus I had to navigate some street/hotel construction. There was no organization or formal waiting line so when a bus arrived, which only occurred sporadically, there was pushing and shoving. I did not get on the first bus but with a little strategic standing did on the second try.

At 7 p.m. the Expo ended and we started heading for the doors to get the return bus. Someone came out to say that the bus had stopped for the evening due to the traffic. Now what – there were no taxicabs and Atlanta was paralyzed. I was tired but people started walking.

They said – go to Building B and maybe there would be taxis. People pretty much dispersed and I walked inside one building after another, toward what I thought was Building B. Going up and down escalators carrying my shopping bag of info I had picked up, I was exhausted. Finally getting outside, I found the Omni Hotel. I figured the bellman could get me a taxi, but not so quick! Atlanta was still packed with people and cars and it took another thirty minutes to get a taxicab. Other conventioneers joined me in the car and we got back to the convention hotel. I headed for the bar to get some wine and dinner. Success! I wasn't leaving that hotel again that evening!

## BUYING SHOES IS ALWAYS A PROBLEM

*Nordstrom's to the rescue!*

My feet are different sizes as everyone's are but the stroke exacerbated it. If my shoes are not perfect, I don't get the proper support for my right foot. Then my ankle turns and it's not safe. The helpful shoe salesmen always try to put the shoes on my right foot, but I have to do it! So, I wind up having to tell them about the stroke – what a drag!

I've found, after going to expensive and not-so-expensive shoe stores, that I get consistently good sales assistance at Nordstrom's. Starting as a shoe store before becoming a department store chain, their shoe department (and others) remains stellar.

It is not uncommon for me to try out ten or twelve pairs of shoes at a sitting. The typical scenario is that after I get each pair of shoes on, Debbie watches as I walk to see if my ankle is turning, or if it looks as though I have decent support. We can easily spend an hour or more trying to buy a pair of shoes or sneakers to no avail. Frustrating for me, Debbie, and the salesman.

I've learned – if the shoes fit and provide the necessary ankle support…buy them at any price.

*They're gold!*

**GETTING OUT OF THE SNOW!**

A coping strategy to live a more independent life and not be reliant on the weather. If you are handicapped and not living in a warm climate – move!

In late 2001, though walking unaided, I still had considerable deficits. Debbie had retired from teaching after thirty years and we moved down to Naples, FL. We had built a small single story villa home in a Country Club community. The thinking was that Florida is handicap friendly and with its flat topography, I would be more independent.

Traveling on business up North, I was and still need to be more cautious with hills and other environmental issues. And I am not comfortable walking in snow or on icy streets. Think the current winter – 2014-2015, I would have been locked in if we were still up North. So Florida solved that concern! Debbie said, *"I was ready for a change and though Bob was independent, not so in bad weather."*

I moved my business interests down to Florida and after about two years of retirement in Florida, Debbie started a tutoring company – A+ Skills Tutoring in Naples (www.AplusSkills.com). As you might guess, she has successfully grown the service over the ten year period.

# CHAPTER 12

# FRIENDLY CHATTER – A SELF-ADVOCACY STRATEGY TO SUCCEED

Isn't everyone friendly? Don't they like to meet new people and learn new things?

*Friendly chatter as a strategy! Friendly chatter as a way to self-advocate! Am I crazy? Am I losing my marbles?* **No** *I'm not! Definitely not!*

When people suffer a stroke or any serious disease for that matter, they are often pissed, angry and sometimes resentful or a combination. I witnessed all of this, and more, during both the three months I was in the nursing home and the years at Main Street in Danbury. These folks were not giving off good vibes. None of this was constructive.

*So yes, friendly chatter as a strategy for success!*

I tend to be a chatty person. It's probably the New Yorker in me. I learned it is extremely helpful when one is navigating the healthcare system on so many levels. Let's start with the phone where Debbie advocated early in my recovery, and I did later. Having been in the call center business, I know that friendly chatter is often helpful when you are speaking with a call center representative. This is particularly so if one is trying to right a wrong, or trying to arrange something difficult.

For example, when one is on the phone trying to figure out something with medical insurance or appointment scheduling, I have learned it certainly helps. The friendly chattiness can result in the rep going the extra mile to solve the problem and thereby achieving a constructive result, where a diffident conversation often results in a negative outcome. And a nasty conversation, even worse!

Just how do I do this? I look for some commonality in our backgrounds, geographies, experiences, or people I might know, or people who are in the public arena. The weather, current events, football, other sports, kids, just something to talk about!

For example, recently I was trying to schedule a neurology appointment. At first blush, there seemed to be no convenient openings. While the appointment scheduler was looking we started chatting about the upcoming weekend. When she came back with the inconvenient times the friendliness allowed me to easily ask that she look again, to which she gladly complied rather than blowing me off. We continued to chat and suddenly she indicated a new, more convenient time. If I was diffident, or didn't push the point, it wouldn't have happened. She said that she was able to reorganize something in the schedule.

○

Friendly chattiness certainly helped me while I was planning our trip to Australia two years ago. Mind you, this is nice, polite and respectful chatter. I was getting nowhere and getting discouraged trying to use my American Airline miles to get two business class seats for our trip. Going in, I knew that this was one of the toughest awards to score in the world. My initial experience bore that out. I would call and there wasn't any first or business class availability. Coach was out due to the trip's length, my physician's advice and Debbie agreed.

One Saturday early in January, I had just about had enough and I thought to myself,

*I am going to give it one more shot.*

I knew of a service that arranges award travel for a fee. That was my Plan B. I was fed-up and ended several calls by doing what I call: a courteous hang-up in which I just nicely explain that we are getting nowhere so I am going to hang up.

Anyway, I got lucky and got a real pro on the phone. My experience just told me so. I told her a little of my stroke story and how we were trying to go to Australia. After listening for just a few minutes she piped in that her dad had recently had a stroke and we talked about him for a few minutes. She was very upset and I immediately stopped talking about me, shifting the conversation to her Dad, sensing my problems could be over! This gal was going to accomplish it.

She said, *"Are you on a speaker phone?"* *"YES"*

She spoke with a southern accent - *"Now you just put me on the speaker and go about your work. I will let you know when you are set."* She asked a few questions as time went by, and started to look at the inventory of the many partner carriers in the ,One World Alliance, not just American and Qantas, the more obvious ones. Incidentally, that's how you can tell the pros.

Low and behold, she had found available seat inventory! And about thirty minutes later, she said the magic words, *"You're all set!"* And we were. Bingo. Next stop – Sydney!

And, as an aside, if you are getting nowhere when talking to a call center representative, just politely end the call. Then call back. The airlines, the insurance companies, the healthcare establishment and most other larger companies have zillions of agents on the phone, so keep searching for a more knowledgeable or cooperative representative. That's part of successful self-advocacy. It's kind of a pain. Just grit your teeth and be friendly to accomplish your objectives on the phone!

◌

Spending all those months, weeks and days doing one therapy or another, I found that becoming friendly with the staff helped me in a number of ways:

**First**, my chatting helped to reinforce in the minds of the therapists my seriousness about the therapy and recovering.

**Second**, by chatting with the staff, the therapists came to understand that I valued them and was sensitive to their interests and lives – not just mine, which as a practical matter made them even friendlier. I also like to think this motivated them to work harder and longer with me which at least some times was true, no doubt about it.

**Third**, a lot of therapy is quite repetitious and boring. At some point I had a mental sanity issue. If nothing else, chatting made the time go faster.

**Fourth**, it provides a way to learn new things about my disease and what was going on around me. The therapists and support staff had a firm grasp of what's going on in the field so by being friendly, the staff often volunteered their information. Nothing confidential, mind you.

⌂

This may all sound trite and I am not bragging. Over the years therapists have often told me that so many of the patients are just going through the motions, that my proactive approach to therapy was refreshing. Whether they were just being nice, it seemed to allow me to stand out from the crowd, which was strategic and at the end of the day, worked. A coping strategy!

*Be friendly and chatty! But be sensitive to the fine line that you don't come off as too pushy. Being chatty and friendly worked for me as a patient, and for Debbie as a caregiver and advocate. It still does!*

# CHAPTER 13
# THE UNSUNG HEROES – THE CAREGIVERS

*Stroke strikes, like a Midwestern tornado suddenly dropping from the clouds. And with it possible deaths, sickness, havoc, and unexpected chaos that someone must clean-up. A mess to fix! Say Hi to the caregiver's role!*

*—Bob Mandell*

Debbie never planned it. She didn't know how to do it. Several times she was under unexpected time pressure. All the focus was on me, the survivor. Yet, make no mistake about it, her life had dramatically changed. Working full-time, she said that she felt like she was in a pressure cooker.

Another lovely woman caregiver in Minneapolis, who is a good friend of my Score mentor, termed it "overload." A gentleman caregiver friend of mine said the toughest thing for him while taking care of his Dad, who had suffered a stroke, was balancing the time he wanted and needed to spend with him and his very demanding career responsibilities.

*The caregiver spouse or partner – the Unsung Hero!*

Debbie's experience was typical. She had a day to accomplish something that she had never done before – getting me into the correct rehabilitation environment. Many others have similar stories.

But there was more than one thing that she had to adapt to - another was legal. Since we each had a living will that was not an issue. However, she needed a Power of Attorney so that she could transact business and legally act as my agent.

A stop at the family attorney to have him draw up the necessary paperwork was in order. Today there are websites that can provide the forms for Power of Attorney. Still!

Knowing little about stroke, since it had never occurred in her family, she had to quickly get up to speed on just what we might be facing in the future. It wasn't good.

Thoughts that went through her mind were
- What kinds of doctors and diagnostic tests would he require?
- What outpatient rehabilitation would he need?
- What would Bob need after his rehabilitation stay?
- What were the insurance and financial implications?
- How would our joint lives change?
- How could she maximize the outcome?
- And many others.

Life cannot completely revolve around the survivor. It's not healthy and productive. While they are providing caregiver services it is important for a person to maintain their outside activities. Debbie did. A recent study published in *Stroke Connection*, the American Heart Association publication, confirms that notion finding that "older, active and confident caregivers were the happiest." It also found that being in better physical health and continuing with hobbies and activities was most helpful to their well-being.

Debbie continued to teach in Greenwich and even kept teaching her Adult Education women's exercise class several evenings a week.

Another study that I found interesting was a study out of Northwestern Medicine which found that the greatest amount of stress for the caregiver emanated not from the patient, but rather from friends and relatives who showed, "a lack of understanding and help." That actually is a threat to the caregiver's own wellbeing. Not good! Second guessing by family members or friends can often be very emotional and destructive. There can also be family tensions in connection with money and long-term financial considerations. All, less than constructive.

An important caregiver role is patient advocacy, which is clearly ripe with emotion. The caregiver and patient want action and results yesterday. Of course they do! Sometimes, Debbie did. Unfortunately, the healthcare system does not always move that fast, causing frustration. We have discovered that finding a way to channel that frustration will ultimately be far more positive.

*Smile and take it easy. This will likely make for easier dealings with the frustrating roadblocks.* **The earlier chattiness chapter holds for the caregiver also.**

Consulting a social worker or a stroke coach and perhaps retaining them on your recovery team might be a helpful adjunct to assist in making arrangements or helping to find helpful resources in a particular community. These folks are knowledgeable about resources that Debbie, the novice caregiver, might be struggling to locate. Debbie consulted with a few social workers, some of whom were a sounding board for questions.

A recent friend, Rob Harris, has published a helpful book, *We're in This Together: a Caregiver's Story* about the caregiver experience. He spends a considerable amount of time laying out the many lessons he learned as he successfully provided care giving services in connection with his dear wife's cancer.

I mention Rob's book which deals with cancer because the principals of the caregiver role in connection with any serious disease are similar. Rob's family situation and the disease details are obviously the differences.

A few of the key points Rob makes in his book and during our conversations include:

- o Patience is a virtue;
- o It's very constructive to make friends with nurses and doctors;
- o There's a fine line between successful advocacy and becoming a nuisance to the staff with possible negative outcomes;

- o It doesn't hurt to ask, but do it respectfully and definitely without an attitude;
- o Stay positive – easier said than done;
- o Play an active role in creating second opinions;
- o Keep positive and optimistic even if it's an act;
- o Be a communicator;
- o <u>You Can Do It!</u>

As all of this recovery effort goes on it is important to maintain as close to normal a routine as possible, a modicum of normalcy. Debbie did that, or at least she tried.

Debbie's personal perspective, *"I had virtually no experience in the caregiver role. Children, yes; but adults, very little! My parents were still alive when Bob had his stroke. The weekend he was meeting my parents, actually Easter weekend, my father lost both of his legs to diabetes. Funny, I remember they got a sample of Bob's cooking, (and one of the reasons I had originally answered his personal ad) – he made this amazing raisin sauce for the Easter Ham, which we all wolfed down. We kept a portion to take to the hospital when visiting my Father, who happily ate some even though he wasn't supposed to.*

*Anyway, my mother really took care of his arrangements, and my father was in the hospital. And later at home, she played the lead caregiver role.*

*So this was all new to me, as I guess, it is with many others. The thing that stands out to me was keeping as close to my normal schedule as possible to maintain my sanity and keep my life going. I kept teaching school and even my adult education woman's exercise classes a few evenings each week. I made it my business to stop by the nursing home every day but I did it when it worked into my schedule. I was never big on bedside stuff so sometimes I would just stay for a half an hour or so. That was fine. I saw him, I kissed him, and made sure things were all right – Bob knew his job was to get better."*

***None of this is easy! A toast to the Unsung Heroes, the Caregivers!***

# CHAPTER 14
# ENJOYING A VISIT TO A BAR

Our telemarketing company was beginning to grow. My business partner, Andy, asked me to go to Wichita, Kansas, to watch the final stages of our new call center site construction and also to oversee the initial recruitment of staff.

This effort was going to take several weeks, so Debbie and I decided to see if we could find a decent rehabilitation facility in Wichita. We found a wonderful center on Rock Road, coincidentally near a first-class fitness center where Debbie could go while I was having therapy.

Before going to Kansas, we had made all necessary arrangements and gotten insurance approval to temporarily transfer my therapy to the center in Wichita. I had made an initial appointment so we were expected.

Arriving at the Nova Care Center,

*"How can we help you in the few weeks that you will be here, Mr. Mandell?"*

I answered, *"Can you get me on a bar stool?"*

The administrator was befuddled and laughed, *"You are kidding, of course."*

*"No, I'm serious. I need to learn how to get on a bar stool. We go out with our employees to thank them for work well done and my first experience last night was totally unsatisfactory. I was sitting on a chair and they were all on bar stools looking down. It just didn't work with me sitting below them!"* And in addition, Debbie and I have always enjoyed hanging out in restaurant bars.

In Wichita, these were talented, dedicated and friendly therapists. After a week or two of routine physical therapy we all held a little meeting.

*"We have the answer, Mr. Mandell. Actually, we have two answers."*

*"We are going to teach you to climb a ladder backwards. And then we are going to see if you can do something else that's a little different."* I was intrigued. Debbie was amused.

They were excited and anxious to proceed. So was I, and most appreciative. First, they rigged a ladder type of apparatus that they used to teach me to climb backwards. I hadn't ever thought of anything like that before but the therapists said:

*"Your rear end movement with the ladder apparatus is the same as climbing onto a bar stool."* Three therapists worked with me over several days during which time they taught me this skill. Struggling, I ultimately started to get the hang of it.

Really, the movement was to get on my toes as best I could and then raise one side of my rear end up in a stretching pattern. Fast forward, these days I use the same movement for other things like getting into high SUV seats and doctor's examining tables. It's a handy move to have. To work in real life at a bar, someone has to hold the stool steady so that it doesn't move while I am getting my rear up. It can be awkward but not if the stool is being held.

When I do this now, Debbie or someone else typically has to either hold the stool or push the stool under the counter with me on it. Otherwise I get on the stool but wind up too far from the counter to be comfortable. A lot of this is dependent on the floor surface. The bar stool moves when it is on tile, smooth wood and concrete. In contrast, when there is carpet, the movement is substantially less. All of these factors are interdependent but impact the result.

*"We have another solution, watch,"* the therapists proudly said. *"I'll bet you have never seen anything like this before?"*

The therapists demonstrated in their kitchenette area. For this technique to work there needs to be a foot rest under the bar counter. Most, but certainly not all bars, have them. I've never been able to deal with a non-foot rest bar area.

"Watch me!" Standing, the therapist put one of her feet onto the foot rest. Then she reached over the bar counter and grabbed the counter from the back to pull herself up with one of her hands. Her second foot then went on to the foot rest. Therapist two, the helper, then pushed the bar stool under the rear of the first therapist who was holding themselves up on the foot rest. Then the therapist let herself down onto the stool, a neat solution with the helper watching that therapist one came down properly on the stool. Voila! Therapist one, was sitting on the bar stool at the bar, and ready for a drink.

Now the therapists said, *"Your turn!"*

I started in a standing position and placed my left foot up on the bar foot rest area. Simultaneously my left hand grabbed over the top of the bar counter and I pulled myself up bringing my right foot to the foot rest. With me now up in the air, Debbie then slipped the bar stool under my rear end, and I let myself down to sit on the stool. She gently guided me down to be sure I was centered on the stool's seat. **A great coping strategy!**

Something to be conscious of, but not necessarily nice - when doing this I learned to cover the inside of my hand with a cocktail napkin before grabbing the back of any bar counters. You can't imagine how many bars are sticky from spilled beer, wine, soda or whatever. I'm not talking about the counter top but rather the back rim of the counter which would be facing the bartender. A patron can't see it, only the bartender. Uuk!

When I don't use a napkin I usually have to wash my hands to get the stickiness off. This means either getting back off the stool and starting over again or getting some water and napkins from the bartender. Either way….. Use a napkin!

But wait, here's a new idea. A gentleman in my writer's group who heard this story said,

*"What about a glove?"* I was surprised and said, *"Great idea, but make it thin. A bulky glove will make it awkward."* You would probably also need a glove bag. A bit more awkwardness! A surgical glove would be best. They are meant to be disposable so can easily be thrown away.

This is all very well and good when Debbie is with me but that's not always the case. If she's not along, I'll ask the bartender, or whomever I am meeting, or a friendly patron to assist in this little process.

In case you are a bit shy or don't like to call attention to yourself, I have never been turned down when I asked for help. Just ask!

*By the way, if you need it, this is a unique ice breaker!*

# CHAPTER 15

# NEW SITUATIONS – THE FIX IS IN

Being handicapped, I often get into situations that require a quick fix. That is particularly the case, being very active.

Several months ago I attended an all-morning public relations meeting that required quickly adjusting to a new venue environment. I drove 45 minutes up to Ft. Myers where the session was to be held, and first the Google Map surprised me by having a small but important error in the directions. I can understand because it was quite confusing.

Interestingly, a few summers ago we saw how Google gathers its data for their maps while we were visiting the Swedish Port of Visby on a cruise ship. A small Google logoed car outfitted with a video camera drove the area, quickly winding around from street to street – in and out. It was interesting to watch for a few minutes until the car disappeared into some non-visible small streets on the Island, which incidentally is a lovely place to visit. It's very calming with many seemingly happy families. We would have liked to spend a few days there – maybe next time.

Back in Ft. Myers, the directions did not take me to the exact location. Google's directions brought me to the entrance of a country club, which, as it turned out, was out of sight but just around the corner from the Government building where the session was to be held. Fortunately, the gate to the Club was attended and the gate attendant correctly directed me to the building.

*I was glad to be early! This is something I always try to do when going to a new location. I can't run to make up time and don't like the pressure of being late, so I allow a few extra minutes. One stroke is enough, thank you!* **That's a coping strategy** *also.*

Entering the government building for the first time, I waved to a few people that I casually knew, shook a few hands and checked in. There were about 75 participants expected.

When I entered the room where the panel discussion was to be held, I entered and was surprised that there were only bridge chairs and no tables to utilize for food or note taking. What a pain! A light breakfast was advertised to be followed by six speakers, likely requiring some note taking. Since breakfast was advertised I did not bother eating anything at home as the session started at 8 a.m.

So here were a few new challenges – eating something for breakfast and note taking with no table. In these instances I quickly size up the situation and try to create a fix which allows me to proceed without being side railed by my handicaps.

So here I am with a few choices – I could leave – nope; I could skip breakfast which means a stomach ache since the meeting was scheduled all morning – again –that isn't going to happen; or a fix, I would just have to hog two chairs and use the second seat as a desk-top.

Frankly, I wasn't real comfortable with the choice since chairs were getting to be a premium as participants streamed in, but that was the only practical answer so I stuck with the best of several bad choices!

As for breakfast, a bagel, coffee a few small pieces of fruit, pretty basic but what I could manage. I carried the food but someone volunteered to get me a cup of coffee while they were getting theirs. Very nice!

And then there was the note taking – I always bringing a hard-cover folio or notebook in case there is no table to lean on. Another coping strategy. I just put the folio on the seat of the extra chair on my left and took notes – the fix was adequate but I hope they have tables next time – it's a lot easier!

And next time, I'll take the time to have breakfast and not leave myself so vulnerable. Then there will be tables – you can bet on it!

◌

Last year I registered for the high-powered Imagine Solutions Conference with a raft of nationally known speakers. When I had contemplated going to the conference, I was very excited about the potential to hear some good ideas and network with people with whom I ordinarily would not have contact.

The morning of the conference I really wasn't in the mood to attend and adapt myself to the new situations that I knew would require accommodations. Debbie even said, *"You don't really want to go today, do you?"* *"You know, I don't feel like being bothered. I'd rather work on the book in my office."*

But I had already paid the registration fees, which weren't refundable, so I reluctantly went. And, sure enough there were about 600 attendees at a local Ritz Carlton hotel, actually in a tent on the grounds. And, as I guessed, I did have to make some accommodations.

When I first heard about the tent it gave me pause. Would it have a floor and would there be air conditioning were just a few of my thoughts! Upon arriving I surveyed the situation as I always do. Thank goodness there was a carpeted floor in the tent and tables and chairs so walking and note taking were not an issue. And the tent was air conditioned, actually too much so.

*I purposely got to the tent a bit early to get an end seat.*

This way, should I have to take a call or use the restroom during one of the sessions my movements would not require climbing over other attendees, which for me is awkward and possibly challenging with my balance issues.

A challenge emerged, since lunch was planned out on the grass. Scoping it out, I realized that I would have to ask for help getting to the tables and chairs. Then I would also require help getting food as the food was being presented in a buffet style line. When there is a buffet line I have learned to take a plate and then find a spot between the food presentation plates to set my plate down so that I can serve myself.

No such luck here as the serving plates were too close. For me, difficult! As people were walking out to the grass, I asked a woman whom I had been speaking with earlier for some assistance. In an earlier life she had been an occupational therapist so I guessed she would be accommodating, as she indeed was. Actually she and her husband were most gracious. We had a most pleasant lunch but only because I asked for help.

It all worked out and I was definitely glad I went to the conference. Frankly, I would definitely prefer to not need all of that assistance but I have learned to ask for help. **Another coping strategy**. Learning to do that has been a tough lesson, particularly when I don't know the people. Men probably have a tougher time with this than women, maybe it's the macho thing.

*But no one has ever turned me down. Ever!*

# Part IV

# *Attitude Therapy*

Never confuse a single defeat
with a final defeat.

*F. Scott Fitzgerald*

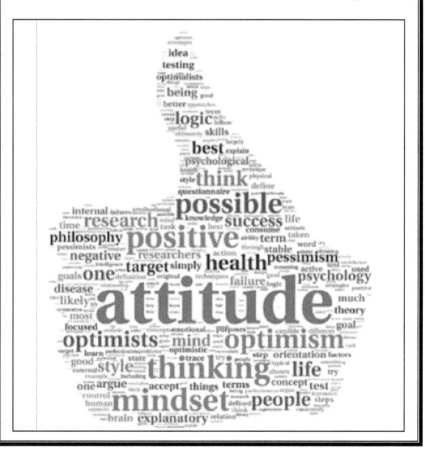

# CHAPTER 16
# SLAY THE GIANT KILLER – DEPRESSION: PART 1

Over the years people often have asked how I avoided depression. **It's a substantial problem post-stroke.** I always answered that I was so sick that I didn't realize the true extent of my condition. However, writing this book, I came to realize that my answer was far too simplistic, and perhaps capricious. I didn't have psychological training and so I wasn't seeing the true reality; I couldn't "see the forest from the trees".

*I have to find the right words to explain how I fought depression.*

To assist me, I enlisted the help of my friend, Udo Fischer, a clinical psychotherapist who was also trained in neuropsychological rehabilitation. He kindly probed me to articulate the true story. As we spoke about my experience one sunny afternoon at a Starbucks in Naples FL, he helped me put into words some of the strategies I had utilized, admittedly unwittingly.

*The first and most important thing I like to call Mindset Strategies.*

**And the first of these was 'Taking on the Challenge,' the challenge of recovery!** Udo emphasized that this was key to my success. In all of the things that I have previously described, I was embracing the process of recovery and though it was difficult, **it was totally doable. YOU TOO!**

For clarity, an alternative way to view this would be to consider the situation from the perspective of intellectual orientation: *taking an action orientation versus, remaining in an intellectually paralyzed stable but non-active state.* I could not have recovered if I had fallen into the trap of intellectual paralysis. And rest assured that trap is devastating to post-stroke lifestyle; for the survivor and as important, the caregiver(s)!

*If I could do it, so can others.*

Taking on the Challenge laid the groundwork for everything else that I accomplished. **If I hadn't taken on the challenge, then I don't see how I would have had the motivation or energy to do the tough stuff and see it through.** I would have faded; just as the nursing home doctor quoted at the beginning of the book told me would happen.

Here, I was sitting in a wheelchair and unable to walk, talk, think or anything else very much. How was I going to do this? My answer to myself - **I WILL!**

According to Udo, this strategy is emphasized by many past and contemporary spiritual teachers, success coaches and Eastern philosophers. You don't have to know in advance the detail, or how exactly you will accomplish success. But **you do have to make a decision that you will be successful and then start to envision that success and finally, more importantly, believe in it.**

*Being caustic, believe your own bullshit, but in this case, the bullshit is real. Make it that way. Make it happen!*

This motivational, envisioning exercise is utilized, as well, in certain psychotherapeutic approaches and finds itself partially expressed in an old mantra taken from cognitive behavioral approaches to treat depression: "Action precedes motivation." **Suspend your disbelief and hopelessness temporarily and take action! The rest shall follow.**

*They'll help. The therapists are eager to help. I can do this.*

So, the most important way that I took on the challenge was to adapt a one step-at-a-time process. I figured I should be able to take a step, just one to get myself going. If I did that, it would have been a successful day. And then I wouldn't get depressed. And it went from there. I've discussed this in more detail in Chapter 10.

As Udo related, this strategy, One-day-at-a-time,' is essential in 12-step approaches for the recovery from any addiction or self-defeating behavior. It is also used in many psychotherapeutic schools. It prevents us from projecting too far into the future and becoming overwhelmed and discouraged when some ultimate goal appears absolutely unattainable given our situation at the moment.

*Make it a game.*

I've learned that recovery can be a slow process so to do it day in and day out, I thought, let's make it a mental game. ***The game - to try to beat yesterday's self.***

First, walking between those parallel bars, aided and then unaided. Then, with a quad cane, aided and unaided, and similarly with a single cane, I was embracing a one-step-at-a-time process. This was later followed by time in a shallow, indoor pool where the buoyancy helped me to gain the mental confidence that I could walk again. And then finally on land without a cane – all a step-at-a-time!

The key was intellectually **embracing that little game with none other than me.** Now, this all took patience, which wasn't a strong suit of mine in my pre-stroke fifties. So the game gave me a way to have little wins on a regular basis to pacify my patience and keep me going.

*Stay in the moment - Stay on today!*

**To play that little game with myself, I had to do just that - Stay in the Moment.** Udo had counseled that this is a way to avoid depression. Anxiety often is triggered by thoughts projecting negative outcomes into the future. Depression is more likely to be triggered by focusing on negative events or experiences in the past and extrapolating from them. So I focused on the current state of affairs.

Not looking back or forward, my emphasis was on today, not yesterday, maybe tomorrow, but not much more.

That thought kept me focused on the here and now. It helped me to avoid looking back to think about the many should have's or not have's. Somehow, I realized that focusing on them would have driven me nuts, with the likely outcome of depression. God was watching!

So Udo said that this process is sometimes called *a regret* orientation. Certainly, in this situation, it was best not to project what my life would have been had I not had the stroke, particularly in those early years.

*It is history and therefore not actionable!*

Here's one; would there, could there, should there have been a better outcome if I had gone to the hospital earlier the night of the stroke when I first called 911. There still is no shortcut fix for a hemorrhagic stroke like I had and, most definitely, wasn't one 19 years ago, so I don't think so. But I'll never know – best not to project. Best not to think about it; it's too depressing.

Several spiritual teachers have elaborated on this wisdom: *"Depression occurs when our thoughts hold onto interpretations of experiences in the past. Anxiety results when we think about potential case scenarios in the future. **Only when we focus our attention on the present moment can we be content**."*

**Only remain focused on what you can do in the here-and-now to improve your situation – nothing else! Focus on the reality of today.**

The strategy that I utilized was to focus on what was the reality. I started to think about different aspects of life and what were the solutions, trying not to think about the problems.

I tried to look at the upside and thought about accepting what I could do with an emphasis on pushing the pencil. Look, the problems could have overwhelmed me, as it does with others, and with it – created severe depression.

In those early times, Debbie played a big role in this by sheltering me from most of the problems, particularly the financial ones.

A final point in this chapter – I've written that I did not personally embrace psychological counseling. However in retrospect that might not have been the best choice.

Stroke being so serious for many and depression so common, counseling might be a better choice in this situation. It certainly gives the patient the opportunity for professional and more objective and non - emotional input unlike that which one might get from friends and family.

# CHAPTER 17
# SLAY THE GIANT KILLER – DEPRESSION: PART 2

*Lifestyle considerations when slaying the giant killer- depression!*

**Udo says lifestyle factors play an important role in avoiding depression.** At the time of my stroke in 1996 I was traveling heavily, mostly out to our telemarketing venture in Lincoln, Nebraska, where my business partner and I shared an apartment. We were commuting nearly every week, which wasn't very easy given the airline connections and Lincoln's relatively limited flight schedule. Though I was exercising at a local Y in Nebraska, I had gained some weight and we were working crazy hours.

### *"Be more caring with yourself"*

That's how Udo summarizes a mental attitude where lifestyle considerations are important. The factors which Udo refers to are regular aerobic exercise, nutritious eating, and good sleep habits. **These are what he calls the *'Three healthy lifestyle pillars.'*** These can influence our emotional well-being more than one would think at first blush.

At both the nursing home, and even more so at Main Street in Danbury, much of my therapy had an element of exercise. Of course my exercise intensity had changed post-stroke and I was starting at a very low level, however, regular exercise still made me feel better, as it does today.

Udo suggests that 80 to 90 percent of mild to moderate mood and anxiety disorders can be alleviated with regular aerobic exercise rather than pharmaceuticals. Maintaining an elevated heart rate is the operable criteria in utilizing exercise to beat depression. And, to be successful, the exercise must be **no less than three or four times per**

**week and definitely more is better.** For my part, I try to exercise every day but as a practical matter, life sometimes gets in the way so five to six days a week is more realistic.

A second lifestyle factor in beating depression is diet. Udo recommended I focus on a Healthy Eating Pyramid via turning the old, traditional Food Pyramid upside down. He says it is best to emphasize high-nutrient density foods. He suggested eating several portions of fruits and vegetables, a few whole grains, if need be, nuts, and more natural, healthy fats. Also oils like avocado, olive and coconut oil, and especially foods rich in Omega-3's, ground flax and hemp seeds, walnuts, algae derived DHA/EPA or some selected high quality, fresh fish oil products. Dramatically cutting down on mass-produced meat, dairy and processed fats are all critical. If you cannot resist meat and dairy ensure you obtain it from organically, pasture-raised and farmed animals.

**Furthermore in a healthy diet one should reduce or entirely eliminate processed and fast foods which are most often full of sodium, sugar and fat with little nutrition or, even worse, toxic additives, steroids and antibiotics.** These foods lead to more inflammation and faster deterioration of your healthy brain tissues, something you definitely don't want after a brain event like a stroke. If need be, work with a specialized dietician who can assess a potential need for dietary changes or supplementation.

At the nursing home, early on, Debbie had arranged for daily fruit salads at lunch and her mother made most of my dinners with an eye to nutrition. Friday nights we cheated. There was a limit! Though this happened gradually, today, I am largely a vegetarian eating large healthy salad, fruits, vegetables and pasta dishes. Most of my cheating is with cheese but I rationalize it with the need for protein.

Finally, getting a good night's sleep is important to recovery. I, and everyone else, needs energy to recover and I learned that energy partially comes from sleep. Unquestionably, sleeping seven or eight hours per day was constructive, particularly in those early years. Some resources recommend even more, closer to nine hours.

## *A new purpose!*

*Fighting and winning at depression, is there a new purpose?*

Yes, I think there is. Today, I try to find meaning in my new situation. I'm still handicapped, though not anything like what was predicted. So, over the last few years I have sought to find new challenges that are conquerable, new ways that I can communicate the upside of my situation.

*Smell the roses, as it were.*

Again, Udo pointed out that this cognitive strategy of mine was rooted in ancient Eastern philosophies and wisdom. Consequently, as he learned in his own clinical studies, neuropsychological patients from the Eastern hemisphere often recover more swiftly and are less likely depressed from strokes or any other types of traumatic brain injuries. They are, by their Eastern cultures and spiritual conditioning, more likely to suspend a very negative evaluation of a dramatic life event since they trust that one cannot predict what the constructive meaning of it might be in hindsight.

It is reminiscent of an old story often being told in Buddhist or Taoist cultures in different variations. Udo remembered that a renowned children's book called '*Zen Shorts*' by Jon J. Muth titles it with '*The Farmer's Luck*':

> "*There was once an old farmer who had worked his crops for many years.*
> *One day, his horse ran away. Upon hearing the news, his neighbors came to visit.*
> "*Such bad luck,*" *they said sympathetically.*
> "*Maybe*", *the farmer replied.*
> *The next morning the horse returned, bringing with it two other wild horses,*
> "*Such good luck! The neighbors explained.*

*"Maybe", replied the farmer.*

*The following day, his son tried to ride the untamed horses, was thrown off, and broke his leg.*

*Again, the neighbors came to offer their sympathy on his misfortune.*

*"Such bad luck", they said.*

*"Maybe", answered the farmer.*

*The day after that, military officials came to the village to draft young men into the army to fight in a war. Seeing that the son's leg was broken, they passed him by.*

*"Such good luck!" cried the neighbors.*

*"Maybe" said the farmer.*

\*\*\*\*\*\*

*You get it!*

*So after each very significant life event and sometime passing, it became clear that those seemingly negative occurrences led to something completely new, different and often rather positive in the long run. For example, in the story, the farmer's son's injury helped him avoid the draft and thereby going into a gruesome war that he most likely would not have survived.*

When my mindset is about new things, about helping others, assisting others to find a way through it, I think, maybe the stroke was a good thing. Friends have said that God gave me the strength to recover, as I have, so that I could help others in a similar situation.

This book, speaking publicly and the research foundation that I, with several others, have created, and will be discussed later, for example!

*Slay the giant killer, depression…with a new purpose, mind games and a healthy lifestyle!*

# CHAPTER 18

# REFLECTIONS ON BEING A VICTOR

*With sensitivity to the realities of stroke, when things get rough,*
*The tough get going!*
*—Bob Mandell*

My friend and Score Counselor (SCORE is a volunteer business counseling service composed of retired executives), Bob Jones, recently re-read these last two chapters about beating depression. He said, *"Do you think you've been very clear throughout the book in defining "Victor" as a frame of mind, an attitude, a recovery mode… something one always is, and not the honor of having won?"*

When Bob speaks that way, I jump *"Maybe not! Let me revisit and be more explicit."*

### So, how to be a "Victor?"

When I think of the term "Stroke Victor" I think in terms of fully embracing one's recovery. **It means doing the best I, or you, can do, given the hand you, or I, were dealt.** We have to embrace the recovery process and then maximize the recovery in relation to the deficits. If, after all the good effort one puts in they still can't walk properly for example, someone is still a "Victor." **It's about the effort, the trying, and the mental engagement that makes the "Victor."** As Bob said, *"it's not the honor of having won"* or, in this case, completely solving the deficit. **It's the positive and proactive attitude about trying. And the "Victor" will keep trying even in the face of disappointment.**

Because "Victors" don't give up easily or maybe, ever, they keep searching for new answers, new techniques, new providers, perhaps new medicines, "a new bag of tricks". They are always vigilant to catch something new, something that they had never heard of or tried.

One recent evening Debbie and I were watching the PBS Salute to Memorial Day and there were stories of several of our returning heroes. They had suffered serious injuries from roadside bombs etc. They had lost limbs and in some cases were disfigured, but there were heartfelt stories of success. **These heroes were creating new lives, "staying in the game." Being Victors!!**

*And if anyone thinks that this was, or is, easy, guess again! So too, with stroke.*

There are folks who will regain their walking or speech but there are others with more serious brain injuries who, no matter what they do, how much therapy they participate in or exercises they practice, cannot achieve the recovery they seek in connection with the particular deficit. **They are still "Victors." They did and are doing their level best to recover.**

***In the context of their injury they are "Victors."***

Permit me to explore some ideas…to get specific, and if I am repeating some ideas earlier expressed, it is by design for emphasis.

1- Udo expressed the concept of envisioning success. From the get- go it never occurred to me that I would not recover. It just didn't. I always envisioned myself getting back to new. So, I put my mind to accomplishing that goal, with no compromise. I thought that I could do it in a year, which admittedly, turned out to be fantasyland. But even as the year turned into years, I continued to believe that I would ultimately achieve that goal. I still do, 19 years later, though I've redefined what being "back to new" means. To me, "Victors" make the most of the hands they were dealt rather than bemoaning the situation. A leaf out of the counsel I received from the Director of the Brain Rehabilitation Center in Gainesville, which will be discussed later.

2- A mental leap of faith is required when one considers that actions precede results. Take fitness and diet, another of Udo's "things." One has to get on the trail of success, staying there before any results are recognizable. Clearly there is an element of envisioning success to propel you away from that dessert table and to a gym to become engaged in an exercise program, no matter how rudimentary at the beginning.

3- It's the propelling towards a positive goal that separates the "Victors" from the victims. Sitting on my butt bemoaning my physical limitations doesn't do it! An example of an action that will precede results is hiring a trainer or going to a gym where a professional can map out a realistic exercise plan, given one's deficits. You will be rewarded if you stay with the program. I have a routine that I do five or six days per week. You too!

4- I have earlier discussed my "One-Step-At-A-Time" approach in Chapter 10. Thinking through the concept of little obtainable goals is really important to being a "Victor." This is all a fragile state since everyone is different and we all have varied tolerances for failure as well as different reactions to less than good news. So why tempt fate? Think it through along with your caregiver, physical therapist, stroke coach or other professional provider to keep a positive slant on events.

5- Focusing on the now helped me from the beginning. But that focus is in the context of envisioning ultimate success. Looking backward has never been a strong suit of mine, which some may say, perhaps correctly, is a weakness. But in this instance it was definitely advantageous. Sitting around bemoaning what if's, or should have's, is depressing and surely can lead to victim status. By focusing on the here and now, my dealt hand, allowed me to avoid those thoughts. I locked them up in a box, not to be reopened until I wrote this book, which, in retrospect, is why I delayed it as long as I could and did. For some who wish to attain the feeling of "Victor," perhaps the lock and key is a worthwhile strategy.

6- One place one definitely wants to use the lock and then throw away the key forever, the negative Mr. Grinch! **Get rid of him or her.** It's so counter-productive. They will get in your way a million times as you recover, or perhaps you won't recover because Mr. Grinch found the key and let him or herself out into the sunshine to screw you, or me.

*So what is a "Victor?"*

It's a frame of mind, an attitude, a recovery mode...something one embraces and always is. It's not the honor of having won because it's a mental game one plays with himself. A self-engagement! And everyone's definition of "the win" is different and highly dependent on the nature of the deficit.

*"Victors" keep themselves "in the game" rather than "throwing in the towel."* And as long as they stay the course, they achieve the best recovery they can.

# WE ALL CAN BE VICTORS!

## Part V

# *Opportunity Knocks*

Surprising results occur but only by
taking the bull by the horns.

*-Bob Mandell*

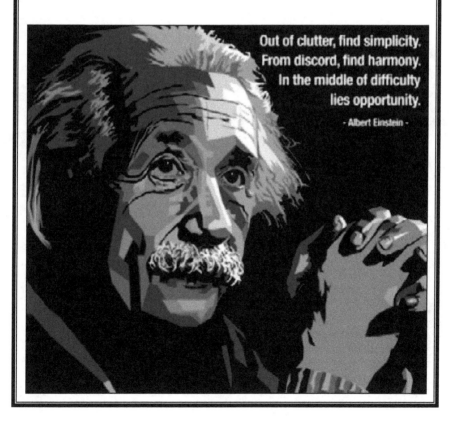

Out of clutter, find simplicity.
From discord, find harmony.
In the middle of difficulty
lies opportunity.

- Albert Einstein -

# CHAPTER 19

# WHAT I WANT IN MY THERAPISTS

Recently I met with a bright young woman, Caryn McAllister, who runs a growing and well-respected boutique therapy company, HQH Therapy, in Fairfield County, Connecticut. She is focused on quality care, a sentiment that certainly rings true with me. That got me to thinking –

*How would I summarize my experiences with therapists, be they physical, occupational, speech or psychological, and more importantly, what led to my best outcomes? And what can we learn?*

I have had many, many therapists, with engagements lasting for years as with Irene in Florida to many months, weeks and also for only 30 minutes. I am paying for these services with cold, hard cash, or through insurance reimbursements, which these days are valuable because they are so limited. That said, I am hyper-sensitive to receiving excellent services and am proactive if the services are not meeting my needs. You too!

As she described her corporate philosophy, Caryn gave me succinct, wise and important perspectives. The pillars of her company are compassion, education and excellence, which are a wonderful start from my patient perspective. There are, however, important considerations in each of these factors that translate into successful patient outcomes.

**COMPASSION**

I realized that I have had the most success with compassionate and friendly therapists. Being sympathetic, they understood that at a relatively young age for a stroke, I had taken a hit and they were supportive of my efforts to recover. I felt like they genuinely cared about my success and worked hard to help me achieve it. They were friendly, caring and sympathetic, but not pushovers so they coached me to excel. With pushovers, who in the name of sympathy or friendliness would allow me to breeze through my therapy sessions, I never achieved anything.

Working with a compassionate person is in sync with my friendly chit-chat philosophy discussed in Chapter 12. But, at the end of the day the coaching/therapy has to be serious.

Conversely, a therapist who is just going through the motions is a waste of time. They are watching the clock or are preoccupied with their own issues or interests. Thirty minutes and only once is my motto.

## EDUCATION

The successful Bill Gates may have been able to get away with dropping out of college, but in medicine I want professionals with degrees from schools that I know about. Schools I am less familiar with simply require extra due diligence and the same if the person was educated offshore since I am not familiar with every school in every geography. For example, Irene, who I will talk about later in the book, was educated in the Philippines, at the best physical therapy program in Manila. Certainly good! What I am not interested in are therapists who have degrees from what I call "University of Nothing," no matter where the school is, no offense intended.

There also is the education one gets from the "school of hard knocks," from their experience. Treating more patients gives the therapist different perspectives and experiences, no two of which are the same.

*My best outcomes have been achieved with experienced people from good schools.*

I've learned that every decent therapist has his or her own techniques, nuances and processes, either learned in school or by their experiences. I call that "their bag of tricks." Although therapy is based on science, from my patient perspective there is considerable art when a therapist is on the firing line, treating a patient, particularly when the issues are not straight-forward.

As a stroke survivor, my issues are best treated by therapists who have at least some neurological training and are knowledgeable about the implications of brain injuries. Do I want a Chevrolet auto mechanic to work on my BMW?

I have been asked just how I find this information.

The answer is: I observe or ask.

Typically in a mid-sized or larger therapy facility, degrees, honors and medical society memberships are not readily available to observe or they may be in a different place than I am. In contrast, smaller or single therapist offices often have their credentials hanging on the wall.

During my first visit, as the therapists are doing their evaluation, I inquire in a casual, friendly manner where they were educated and what their degrees and specialties are. Have they had neurological courses and experience with diseases of the brain? Do they have experience with stroke patients and how have they impacted those patients?

Since most patients don't ask these kinds of questions, I am interested to see their attitude about my questions and how they handle the answers. Embracing my questions is a good sign, a callous attitude or not taking me seriously, is not.

## EXCELLENCE

You would think that excellence is kind of a given, but in reality it's sadly not. But this is what makes Caryn's practice so successful. She spends a considerable portion of her time recruiting the best therapists. And from my observations, there are relatively few therapists who are truly excellent. So it's not such an easy job.

So what is this thing called excellence? It is a mindset. It is delivering the finest services available. It is motivational. A mantra: **I refuse to take no for an answer.** Rather, we will find a creative solution for the patient's betterment. It is the intellectual curiosity to keep moving in a positive manner and to care enough to look into another's "bag of tricks" for a solution if I don't have one. It's a mindset to go the extra mile, to do the extra research or thinking, to spend the extra time.

When Debbie was teaching in Greenwich, she worked in an elementary school which was all about excellence. If you drove by the school at 5 p.m. or later you would see the teacher's cars in the parking lot even though the school let out at 3:15. The staff was putting the extra time in to develop special programs and lesson plans, an atmosphere of excellence. And they weren't being paid extra for working late. Though they should have been.

*I want to work with people who have excellence as a mindset and then deliver on the promise!*

**Having the best therapists has been one of my ways of beating the odds after stroke –an extremely important game changer.**

# CHAPTER 20

# A PERSONIFICATION OF THE THEORIES AND A CONTRAST

*Turning Caryn's pillars of therapy success into practical reality is the key to succeeding.*

Recently I have been recovering from a fall that I suffered in which I fractured the humerus bone in my shoulder. Why am I talking about a humerus bone injury in a book about stroke? The same mindset that I use for stroke recovery works for nearly every medical issue, only the medical details are different!

It had come time to start physical therapy so I asked the surgeon for suggestions as to therapists. Initially he was a bit reticent about specifics. He made a few general suggestions ... so I said in a friendly, chatty manner, "Being post CVA, my situation is more complicated than your typical injury. This is particularly so since the injury is on my affected side. **If it was you, or in your family who would you go to**?" He thought a minute and then made three suggestions by name.

Self-advocacy to succeed! This is what I am referring to when I make reference to the "The Self Service Model of Healthcare," to be discussed in Chapter 41.

I immediately contacted the conveniently located Physicians Regional Therapy Center and arranged appointments with one of the recommended therapists, Katie Rusk. All of the appointments would be with the same therapist, no team approach here, which I appreciated. In a past therapy engagement for my back at a different therapy center they tried to schedule me using a team approach.

*To my way of thinking **continuity of service is very important**, so I want to work with one therapist for a particular issue.*

During the evaluation visit I immediately appreciated the wisdom of the surgeon's recommendation. Katie was friendly, bright and efficient so she made time to begin treating my arm during the evaluation visit. She was sympathetic to my situation but intent on getting things done, some of which were pretty painful.

Well educated, she had graduated with a DPT from The University of Miami Physical Therapy School, a well-rated program. She also had neurological experience and training, which the therapist who had treated my back did not have. In fairness, it wasn't so important when treating my back.

During the second visit she gave me exercises to do on my own. Without being asked, she provided a reminder sheet describing the exercises. In my last engagement, I had to ask for the reminder sheet, which was then provided.

Since I was in a friendly situation, I started to describe this book to Katie and what I was trying to accomplish. We talked about clinical research and integrative therapies as she pulled and rotated my arm. It was better to talk than scream!

Katie was traditionally educated so she was not familiar with several of the integrative therapies that Irene had exposed me to and I will be discussing later. However, she was extremely interested in learning. More than a casual interest, she was keen to read drafts of the chapters. I was impressed by her interest! She kept pulling!

*Remember Caryn's pillars, compassion, education and excellence.*

*This is the real life experience!*

# CHAPTER 21

# HOW TO KEEP THE THERAPY GOING WHEN THE INSURANCE ENDS

When we were traveling a few months ago, we met an entrepreneurial woman who told us a story of assisting her Dad with the after effects of a stroke.

Her Dad suffered a serious stroke and had burnt through his Medicare insurance-allotted rehabilitation treatments. That isn't too hard these days. So this creative woman spent a few hundred dollars and hired a physical therapist to teach her how to work with her father. She realized that much of rehabilitation therapy is doing various stretches, exercises and repetitive tasks to rewire the brain. Once the therapist had coached her, she visited her father every day to keep progress moving. Working daily, she saw progress and continued her treatments for quite some time.

This tender story made me think – there are many families that could do the same and I thought that it was worthwhile to share this story of family love and success.

There could also be many variations since, like me, not everyone has this kind of family geographic closeness. In my case, none of my children live in Florida, and for others, they have no family at all.

I have been thinking that I might hire a well-trained personal trainer to work with me after my insured rehabilitation runs out. My out of pocket cost will be substantially less than going to a rehab center and doing similar things.

Or one might hire a physical, speech or occupational therapist to work after hours. I am sure that many therapists would be responsive in order to make a little extra money. One can post for jobs available on Craigslist, which allows you to focus on the appropriate geography. Or look for referrals from friends or people in the medical community.

Since therapists don't get paid that highly, I am sure that this is a good way to identify candidates. Paying cash could also help!

*Being proactive to keep making progress is the Victor approach. Letting insurance reimbursement solely dictate your therapy regimen is not!*

*There are lots of iterations if one is motivated. A little creativity could go a long way!*

# CHAPTER 22

# REMARKABLE RESULTS FROM A FAMILY DINNER

*"Opportunities come infrequently. When it rains gold, put out the bucket, not the thimble."*

*—Warren Buffett*

*Of course, Mr. Buffett was referring to financial investments. I am talking about investing in you, in your recovery. **"Put out the bucket to succeed in your recovery by searching for something new, something different, a new path to achieve a Big Blend."***

*—Bob Mandell*

Reading through this manuscript during the editing process, I suddenly had a Eureka moment:

I have not explicitly explained a life-changing concept of mine—

## The Big Blend!

An anecdote to help: When I was a lad growing up on the Grand Concourse in The Bronx, New York on Sunday evenings, our family, like many others in our neighborhood, would walk a couple blocks to one of the Chinese restaurants on 170th Street for a family dinner.

Upon being seated at the modest neighborhood restaurant a waiter would immediately bring a pot of hot Chinese tea to the table, a tradition at these meals. The tea was the lubricant of the meal.

In my anecdote sipping tea or any beverage is addressing post-stroke depression. Just as with the tea which we sipped throughout the meal, depression must be addressed and controlled throughout the recovery. If I didn't have the tea I would not have enjoyed the dinner.

Similarly, if depression isn't addressed the recovery will most likely not go very well. Keep drinking your tea - I did!

In addition to the tea the waiter would, early on, bring a ceramic bowl full of white rice with a metallic top to keep it warm. The rice is typically eaten along with the food which was to follow. In the medical analogy the rice is partaking in physical fitness on a regular basis during the recovery and going forward. The rice is eaten with the dinner as it unfolds. So too, fitness is an important component to recovery as it unfolds.

So to the dinner! There would be a large menu consisting of soups, appetizers and then entrees in two lists, Column A and Column B. We would get to choose a soup, an appetizer and then one or several entrees from each list, to be shared family style. After dinner we would each get to choose our own small dessert.

In my analogy: the soup is the medical evaluation. The medical evaluation gives the medical professionals the basis to design a treatment plan, a base for recovery. So too, the soup provides the base for the dinner. Typically we had Wonton soup though occasionally, Egg Drop soup if my mother got her way.

After a short wait the next course would be served which was the appetizer. For appetizers we would have Egg or Spring Rolls unless my parents wanted to spring for the upgrade to Spare Ribs. In our analogy the appetizer is the feedback from the medical evaluation.

Certainly the feedback is very important and provides a treatment plan for the rehabilitation recovery. The physician and/or the therapists identify which of their techniques will provide the basis for the treatment. So too, the appetizer also sets the stage for the largest course of the dinner, the entrées.

Now, on to the entrees! Our family would eat one or several dishes that we had ordered from Column A. These included Shrimp with Lobster Sauce, Lobster Cantonese or Beef with Broccoli, among others. In Column A of our analogy are the many traditional and well researched techniques that the therapists can use to help the patient improve their functionality and hopefully get better. One or several therapies would be utilized.

But wait! We still had other entrees coming, those from Column B. Typically we would have Fried Rice, Chow Mein, Egg Fu Young, or vegetable dishes, among others. They were an important part of the entire dinner and one not to be skipped to have the full dinner.

In our medical analogy, Column B consists of integrative therapies and other innovative but less researched techniques. Many consider these types of therapies to be non-traditional and not well researched which in many cases is true. So they are not considered. However, they can be very important to the recovery, as they were for me. **In addition, these aren't necessarily included in the traditional medical feedback or considered in the traditional recovery plan.**

Last was dessert. Do I have room – of course! I did like the sweets. I usually had a small scoop of ice cream. I then poured the sweet sauce from my parent's kumquats over the ice cream.

In my medical analogy, dessert is participating in clinical research to get a shot at cutting edge medicine at no cost. How sweet it can be!

**NOW HERE IS THE MESSAGE (and it's a really important lesson)**

**My dinner was not complete without eating all of the courses. And**, I only got satiated if I consumed all of the courses and drank the tea.

**So too, stroke recovery!**

**My, and for that matter, your Stroke Recovery efforts will not be complete without, at least, trying all of the courses, all of the opportunities! So I am suggesting that besides the traditional therapies in Column A, one make choices from Column B and**

look into integrative therapies and then be sure to have the dessert -participate in clinical research.

Based on my experience, the best recovery outcomes, certainly mine, occurred as a result of blending traditional medical approaches, therapy, etc. with integrative, non-mainstream, and little known innovative therapies and techniques and then to top it off, being a participant in targeted clinical research.

This is a case where one and one makes three!

### The Big Blend!

But to do The Big Blend properly, you have to know about the alternatives and understand the elements and opportunities inherent in participating in clinical research. Then you can blend them with the traditional.

*What are they? Where are they? What? What?*

## That's where this book comes in.

With this introduction, let me make an unequivocal statement –

I would not have achieved the recovery that I have without wholeheartedly embracing the concept of the Chinese Dinner - supplementing traditional medicine with supplemental integrative therapies and then participating in clinical research! Each played an important role in my recovery.

Without embracing this systems approach to recovery...

> This book would not have been written;
> If you have heard me speak publicly, that would not have happened either;
> And if you think Debbie and I would have been able to plan and execute an independent trip to Australia and New Zealand with 18 flights, guess again.

**I understand that the reader might think that I am repeating myself, but there is a reason - it's really important!**

**And just an extra note of respect to the traditionalists - in no way do I deprecate traditional approaches. Absolutely not!** (Remember, they were in column A of our Chinese dinner.)

**Traditional medicine got me a long way and put me in a position to successfully take advantage of these other options. And clinical research played an important role in supplementing these therapies, as I will next describe.**

In the next several chapters in this section of the book and the following section – Knowledge is Power; I will be describing the opportunities I experienced with the clinical research process and several innovative and integrative therapies and techniques that I tried. Most worked for me, some remarkably! Others didn't as I will tell you. Other people may have other outcomes and there are no doubt therapies that I have not yet tried. **I am searching for more innovative therapies to share with my community.**

So, this treatment of clinical research and little known therapies is not meant as an exhaustive list of everything that might be out there. These are things I did, or am doing. As I have said before, *"I'm always learning, and there is always something new, or new to me."*

**What's important is to be on the look-out - in the game!**

Stroke recovery, and life itself as we all know, is a work in progress.

So with that…

# CHAPTER 23

# HELPING YOURSELF AND MANKIND BY PARTICIPATING IN CLINICAL RESEARCH

In this changing healthcare environment it pays to be both creative and proactive in order to beat the odds with any disability or illness! It is a must if there is a desire to be a Victor. But this is a case of easier said than done.

*So, where to turn?*

One of the purposes of this book is to make constructive suggestions as to where proactive readers can obtain healthcare from alternative and non-traditional sources. Let's examine a-not-so obvious way of beating the odds at little or no cost.

Progress in healthcare comes from experimentation and researching new ideas and theories. At a certain point in their development efforts, scientific researchers require volunteers like me to participate in their research studies. **The idea is to see if the scientists' theories, when tested with humans, are supported by positive real-life outcomes.** It's an expensive and complex process involving many years of research. There is trial and error and experimentation, followed by additional years of seeking the regulatory approvals to allow the marketing of new medicines or treatment protocols.

From my perspective as a patient, the medical community, for whatever reason, has not done a very good job of managing and explaining this process and the patient opportunities available to the public, at large. I find this remarkable since it is the basis of long-term growth in many segments of the healthcare industry. In any event, the vast majority of the public does not appreciate this process or its opportunities. I didn't! *I only learned about clinical research by accident. A story I will tell later!*

And why would I know about this unless a physician or other healthcare professional took the time to explain it to me, at least introduce it. Today, how many physicians have the time to sit with you to explain this complicated process? Darn few. And it's not their fault – they are under serious time pressure.

When I talk to people about being a participant in clinical research, I often sense a general lack of knowledge and hesitation. People have said things like they don't want to be a guinea pig. Or it's a waste of time or it takes too much time or it doesn't work or friends got injured or other negative comments. Others have said that they had no idea why they should do it, how to access these studies, what is involved and what their commitment would be.

These attitudes come from a general lack of understanding of the process, fear of the unknown and not having their expectations managed properly if they were in a study. When I describe my experiences, my friends seem interested but I am not sure if it is out of anything more than politeness. And when a person harbors negative or questioning attitudes, it takes time to properly address those concerns.

*With that said, permit me to bridge the gap in order to show how a patient can be helped.* How I was helped.

Let's start; this process is called clinical research. There are many institutions and corporations who conduct this research. A great deal of work is funded and/or conducted by various agencies of the Federal Government such as The National Institutes of Health (NIH) or the National Institute of Neurological Disorders and Stroke (NINDS). **With stroke, the government funds most of the research, either directly or indirectly**.

The largest private stroke funder in the US is the American Heart Association through its affiliate the American Stroke Association. Unfortunately, in spite of their good work, it is not nearly enough considering the size and complexity of the stroke problem.
(In the Afterword section appearing later in this book, I will describe

a new private stroke research funding initiative that I am spearheading too address the underfunding of stroke prevention, rehabilitation and recovery research.) THIS IS A BIG OPPORTUNITY!

Other research sponsors include pharmaceutical and other healthcare companies, medical device companies, large research and teaching hospitals and, in some cases local hospitals and medical practices. Often, in the latter cases, the practice or hospital may be funded by the government or one of the larger healthcare companies.

As I see it, there are academic studies and commercial studies. The Gainesville program that I participated in and will describe tended to be academic in nature, at least the studies with which I was involved. Those studies often resulted in academic papers, which might be published or presented at a medical meeting or convention, and also used for further research.

In contrast, the spasticity study that I participated in was being implemented by a neurological practice in Boca Raton, but funded by a pharmaceutical company in France. It is a Phase Three FDA study, which is part of the FDA approval process. This is a commercial study.

When a patient participates in clinical research, they are lending themselves to a research team in return for free medical care, leading edge and state-of-the-art pharmaceuticals, medical equipment, services or techniques that might help them. A subject may also get some compensation or at least expense reimbursement, as I did for participating. I got $ 125.00 per visit as expense reimbursement.

*A fair question is just how is this process implemented in real life?*

When the scientists have completed enough successful research and perhaps conducted animal trials on a particular question or prospective drug, it is time to conduct a human trial. The researchers will determine the specific characteristics of the patients for the study. Criteria could include such things as patient age, symptoms and conditions, among others. It can be quite detailed. The bottom line is, there are many variations depending upon what's being researched, the disease and the stage of research.

Once a study has been designed and panel reviewed there is a need to find participants through a recruitment effort. That may entail working with a local medical practice like the neurological practice in Boca Raton, or a research hospital like I was involved with in Gainesville.

Another neurological practice I am friendly with, this time in Connecticut, was part of a research team that a sponsor organization was using to find patients. They advertised and sort doctor referrals. They also listed their study in one of several clinical research databases that I will describe later.

Similarly, the folks in Gainesville also have a recruiting effort, but as an aside they I believe they struggle to find patients who meet their research study criteria because they have geography against them. Gainesville is a relatively remote college town where mostly young people reside.

***There could be a patient opportunity here!*** *Go to the website* *www.brrc.research.va.gov/*

**There are similar programs at every teaching hospital throughout the nation. These are all opportunities for proactive patients and their caregivers.**

Online, there is considerable general information regarding clinical research. If, like me, one wants to participate in clinical research you have to go in with your eyes open. Before I went into the Gainesville program the director explained to me during the screening process that some of the research helps some patients, but much of it doesn't since it is experimental and doesn't work. My experience confirmed that. Luckily, my major studies worked out very well, but others not at all, at least as far as I was concerned.

**None had a negative impact. This is important.** In my mind the constructive outweighed the unsuccessful hence I'd do it again in a country minute.

**My attitude is that if you don't give it a try you are, in effect, assuming that nothing constructive will come of the research. In my experience that is definitely not the case.**

*If you want to be a Victor, give it a shot - try being a participant in clinical research! Indulge in the dessert I mentioned during your Chinese meal.*

# CHAPTER 24

# AN AHA MOMENT – THE GAINESVILLE STORY

*Here's a perfect example of why I don't keep my hard work a secret. You just never know who is watching or listening but this might never have happened...*

The year was 2004 and we are in Florida. One day a young therapist who had recently graduated from the University of Florida Physical Therapy Program approached me saying, "The way you put yourself into your therapy Mr. M., you should contact the Brain Rehabilitation Research Center at the VA Hospital (BRRC) up in Gainesville where I went to school. See if they would be willing to let you participate in any of their studies." She went on, "They conduct government-funded research and I heard that they always need research subjects – you should see if you would qualify."

Being a subject in clinical research! Aha, now that was new and exciting.

*I never thought of it, had never done it and didn't know what it entailed. I didn't know anyone else who had ever done it. Was this dangerous, scary or could it have negative outcomes? Was this a waste of time and travel money?*

***Or, more positively*** *could this be helpful so that I could make some significant gains?* These and more are the things I considered.

After a pleasant call to Gainesville, a clinician sent me an extensive packet of forms to be completed regarding my stroke and subsequent issues. Soon thereafter a member of the BRRC staff conducted an initial phone screening to see if I might qualify. For my part, I wanted to know what, if any, were the risks and what would I be expected to do. In addition, I needed to determine what kind of time commitments I might be asked to make.

Since a drive to Gainesville is about four hours, I wanted to get a sense that this was not in vain, that I might succeed in getting accepted to the program and that I actually wanted to do it. As usual, I wanted the warm and fuzzy. It did cost time and travel money! It did not appear that the Gainesville program was going to reimburse my expenses.

A few weeks after submitting the forms, and my medical records, and after another phone screening, I was invited for a comprehensive interview and evaluation which was to last a day and a half. (It has been shortened to half of a day now for patient convenience.) Along with their other paperwork was a list of area hotels that offered discounts for BRRC participants. I chose the Hilton which is adjacent to the University of Florida campus. Convenient!

Arriving late in the afternoon the day before my big day and I proceeded to get lost on the huge University of Florida campus. I was doing a dry run for the morning, which is what I have learned to do. I didn't want to be late or in a tizzy from getting lost as I would have without the dry run. I was excited and a bit nervous and there were no GPS's in those days!

During the day and a half screening several staff members conducted interviews focused on their particular research interests. My gait, walking speed, body flexibility and hand/shoulder movements were observed, measured and recorded. I was sliced and diced!

Not only were they interested in my body, but also my mind! I was given several speech, memory recall and cognitive evaluations to determine my intellectual capabilities. These all were to be utilized to determine my appropriateness for inclusion in future studies, of which there were many. I had difficulty with the memory tests which was viewed positively as the researchers needed lower functioning participants. That was the first time in my life that it was good to be lower functioning!

*It was good to be more challenged. Now, that's a new one!*

From personal investigations I've conducted, I learned that rigorous benchmark screening is typical of clinical research. It is necessary so that the researchers are assured that each subject meets defined study criteria. Without it there are no valid or reportable results.

The afternoon of the second day I had the privilege of meeting the Director of the BRRC who reviewed the Center objectives and how I would be chosen for their research studies. He also discussed the facts of life of neurological research.

*"Bob, you have to understand that it is often best for stroke patients like you to learn compensation strategies since you probably will not attain complete restoration of some of your lost abilities. Much of our research focuses on nuanced compensation. It seems to me that you have already done some of that. Your backward walking of stairs without a banister is a perfect example. We were interested to watch that."*

As our meeting was coming to a close, he indicated with a smile that I would be accepted into the research program.

*I was ecstatic. Aha – I can make some serious gains. I have a shot!*

As I was leaving to return to Naples that afternoon, the staff let me know that I would promptly be hearing from them regarding several studies for which I qualified. I happily stopped at Starbucks to get a shot of Joe for the four-hour drive home.

# CHAPTER 25
# MAKING PROGRESS DOING CLINICAL RESEARCH

Having been accepted and scheduled for several shorter studies, I journeyed up to Gainesville as a matter of good faith. I was rewarded. While there, the staff inquired if I would be willing to return for two solid weeks to do a study called "Constraint Induced Therapy (CI)." I was considered a good candidate. As with most of the research studies, I had never heard of it. "Definitely yes," I answered.

Historically and in patient speak, it was traditionally thought that a stroke killed the patient's affected brain cells. Dr. Edward Taub, at the University of Alabama (www.taubtherapy.com), however, made a fundamental breakthrough finding that a stroke did not necessarily kill the brain cells; rather the brain attack shocked some cells into a recoverable coma or sleep. And in any event, the brain could make new connections, essentially rewiring it.

Dr. Taub showed that by bombarding the brain with active stimuli to the affected limb, brain cells could find new pathways resulting in improved limb functionality. However, to be effective this sensor bombardment had to be intensive, lasting many hours per day, over at least a two or three-week time period. Different researchers have tested various numbers of hours per day and intensities. The more intense the better!

Most of the constraint therapy studies focused on the upper limbs, the arm, shoulder, and hand combination. As a cue, to take the unaffected limb out of the equation during this therapy, the subject wears a glove or mitt over their unaffected hand to facilitate concentration on the affected hand. That's what I did. In Gainesville I wore a white cloth glove similar to a catcher's mitt which could only be removed to eat and for bathroom functions. I wore it for a minimum of eight hours per day over the two-week period. While their study methodology was very intensive, it did not require homework. I was there for the full eight hours each day.

In Gainesville, we played all kinds of games; Connect 4, Checkers, Scrabble, cards, and marbles using only the affected hand. We had to do something to constantly use the limb and also deal with the boredom.

While I was in Gainesville during the two week period, to get more bang for the buck, I tried, haltingly initially but more successfully later, to eat my oatmeal at breakfast with my right hand though no one asked me. I figured – the more practice, the better, which worked.

An anecdote! One evening during the first week I went out for an early Olive Garden dinner and decided to try to eat with my right hand. I didn't do the mitt bit, so as not to get it dirty. Being early in the study I was definitely struggling. The waitress first served me water which I promptly spilled and then white wine, which I also spilled. I didn't dare go for red wine, my preference, with all of the spilling. This happened several times until the restaurant manager came over to make inquiries. I told him that I was doing research across town at the Veteran's Hospital and that I was trying to get my right hand to function properly.

He sat down with me for a few minutes and we chatted while he watched and then chuckled. He told me that I could use my right hand as much as I liked and not to worry about the spills – a true gentleman! I appreciated this, but was feeling self-conscious as the restaurant by now was getting busy, so I called a halt to my little experiment.

When I had lunch the following day with the research staff, they were hysterical over my experiment. They wanted to know what manager was so accommodating. But a point had been made! This incident created a "special bond" with the research staff!

*They probably thought I was crazy, maybe, you too!*

**I have told this story for a reason – if you want to win at therapy - go the extra mile and try to create that "special bond." Find a way. It always seemed to help me, sometimes in quite intangible ways! It certainly was an ice breaker and made for a friendlier atmosphere.**

CI was a big win! I relearned to hold a wine glass, which is very important in networking-happy Naples, Florida. Now I can have a passed hor d'oeuvre rather than just drinking. Additionally the improved functionality allows me to cut steak with a knife, eat mussels, and do other things including typing.

*A definite win!*

Today, CI has matured and is practiced clinically in many centers across the nation, in addition to the Universities of Alabama and Florida. I think it is important to go into this with reasonable expectations; CI is not "a walk in the park." I'm not saying it shouldn't be done since it works. Just be prepared for a boring and intense experience.

Let me add another personal observation about CI although others may take issue with me. The therapy staff at a Naples hospital heard about my experience in Gainesville, and asked me to become involved with an out-patient CI program that they had designed. Because it was only 45 minutes per day three days a week, I was very leery about it. To be fair, the Naples therapists did assign homework but the experience was nothing like the concentration I had experienced in Gainesville. I didn't make any additional gains in that study. I may have been a bit burned out and not the greatest subject.

Founder Dr. Taub's writings bear me out; from his website –

*"One of the reasons CI is more effective* (with us) *than other therapy programs is because of its intensity. Patients must also complete exercises independently in the evenings and on weekends."* With CI you get out what you put into it.

*More opportunities in Gainesville by being proactive! This time, a more exploratory study!*

While I was in Gainesville a different researcher, Ned I think his name was, asked me if I was willing to do an exploratory study that they had never conducted with a stroke patient. They called it locomotion training. The study was about speed of walking as it related to body weight. Ned, who was a PhD candidate, thought that two weeks was a good measure.

In this study I walked on a body-weight supported treadmill. I was suspended from a harness to reduce my body weight to various levels. In the early days of the study, the harness substantially reduced my walking weight to roughly half of my actual weight. During the two weeks my walking weight was gradually increased until I was walking full weight during the last few days. A short video of me in the study is on my website www.strokevictor.com.

When actor Christopher Reeves had his terrible horse riding accident there were pictures of him on a similar piece of equipment. He too, was desperately trying to recover before he passed away.

Another win! My walking speed increased by about 25% during the two week period, based on pre and post testing. *I think that was pretty darn good!*

Enough, all of this attention by trained researchers and therapists for free except possibly travel expenses! *I'll say it again; to me, participation in clinical research is a win-win-win situation!*

*Mankind was helped, research science moved forward, and I made some excellent progress.*

# CHAPTER 26

# 2014 – HOW TO FIND RELEVANT STUDIES FOR YOU

That's history. Now let's turn to more current events! During the latter part of 2013 and 2014 with my arm spasticity still an issue, and in the book writing phase, I thought,

*Let's see what's out there that can help. What can I learn, can I improve?*

I began my search on the internet. Since I was looking for research having to do with stroke, I first turned to the relevant stroke associations to see if they could offer some help. The two primary groups are the American Stroke Association (www.strokeassociation.org) and the National Stroke Association (www.stroke.org). Both Associations are primarily focused on stroke prevention, risk factors and education, all obviously very important.

The American Stroke Association does itself fund some research, a good thing. However, neither of their websites had any resources for a survivor looking to find clinical research opportunities. Interestingly, until recently the National Stroke Association had a consumer friendly outsourced service that I personally used but is no longer available. Unfortunate, since it was really helpful to the lay population.

As I continued to look, I came upon My Clinical Trial Locator – www.myclinicaltriallocator.com. It was referenced in a magazine article about clinical research (mentioning me) in Newsmax Magazine, 3/15. The free locator service lists studies for all diseases on a worldwide basis. I did a search for "stroke" studies using the criteria of a test center within one hundred miles of Naples, Fl. The search came up with over twenty studies which were in the recruiting phase, most of which were on the high side of the mileage range.

That there weren't a lot of studies in Naples is not surprising because the Naples area is not a research oriented location. What I had difficulty with was that the results used very clinical terms and therefore I think most families would have difficulty determining if the research was appropriate for their patient. A did a second search using "stroke rehabilitation" that came up with no studies.

**If one were going to use this service I would consider doing the search with the help of a medical professional. At a minimum they could assist with the terminology.**

Believing no stone should be left untouched and continuing to seek opportunities, I **do not rely on any one service or data base**. While this results in some redundancy it also can unearth some relevant research not otherwise located.

That said, I have registered with many clinical research databases including the following:

1- www.ClinicalConnections.com. First, I signed up for their Alert Program. Then I also searched their database for stroke, cardiac and neurological conditions. I did a broad search because under certain circumstances I might be willing to travel out of my geography. I also conducted a narrower search by putting some geographic criteria into the search.

The site has information on the clinical trial process. Click on the Patients and Healthy Volunteers tab along the top and to view the material. Then click on the little arrow under "About Clinical Trials". They also have a short video that gives additional information about the process.

2- www.CenterWatch.com. Again, I registered for their Patient Notification Service. I also checked their data base by first going to Clinical Trials along the top of the site and then clicking on Search Clinical Trials. As with Clinical Connections, the site has descriptive information regarding the process.

3- The US Government site www.ClinicalTrials.gov also has considerable material regarding clinical trials and how to find them. This site is a service of the U.S. National Institutes of Health. **This is a definite must read for anyone contemplating participation in clinical trials.**

When I was writing this chapter the site claimed information on over **150,000 studies with site locations in all 50 states and 185 countries.** Of course, these studies cover all medical issues and maladies. Still that's a lot of studies! Some are relevant to stroke.

The home page has appropriate tabs which bring the reader to quite a lot of detailed and relevant information. For example, they have an extensive explanation of how to find research.

I used the search function on the top right, putting quote marks around many terms with multiple words in addition to stroke. For example, I also used the terms "stroke rehab," "stroke rehabilitation" and "after stroke." When I put "after stroke" into the database I found references to 300 studies with their descriptions and their status. Some were active, others closed. Certainly some could be helpful! As mentioned earlier, there was some redundancy to my other searches. So what!

4- Another government site is www.nih.gov/health/clinicaltrials/ which also comes from The National Institutes of Health. The home page has many links to the clinical trial process and how to find studies. Another excellent resource!

5- A further government site to review is Medline Plus www.nlm.nih.gov/medlineplus/ which is a website for patients and the general public. This is more of a general information site, not a database. Actually, the National Library of Medicine is behind this site. It offers information on diseases, conditions and wellness issues in understandable language.

It also tries to be up to date on medical issues and offers health information. They have a detailed series of information alerts. I signed up for information about clinical trials and a long list of stroke and brain related issues. To get more information on the site click on Senior's under the About Your Health area in the middle of the page and you will find that Stroke is a subcategory. They also had a sub head for clinical research.

6- Another NIH governmental site is the National Institute of Neurological Disorders and Stroke. NINDS funds research across the spectrum from basic research aimed at understanding normal brain and nervous system function to large Phase III clinical trials to test or compare treatments. To access their studies go to www.ninds.nih.gov/. This Institute has clinical trials for many brain maladies including stroke.

Click on "Join a Clinical Trial at NIH" and then click on Stroke and Vascular Diseases. This brings you to the Patient Recruitment Page. As an example of what can be found, I recently found the following NIH resource:

**Stroke and Vascular Disorders >> Acute Stroke**

**General Study Procedures:**
The research studies listed below were open for enrollment at writing time for adult subjects. These studies are being conducted at the Washington Hospital Center and Suburban Hospital. Their research includes use of magnetic resonance imaging (MRI) to study the effects of acute stroke, and experimental treatment of stroke. Please see the links for the procedures and eligibility criteria for specific studies. **There is no cost for participation or for any tests associated with the research.**

**Studies Actively Recruiting Patients:**
Natural History of Stroke: Cause and Development

**For more information about participating in these studies, please contact :**

For protocol 01-N-0007
Lisa Davis, R.N, MSN
CCRC Section on Stroke Diagnostics, Stroke Branch
NINDS Bldg. 10, Room B1D733
10 Center Drive
MSC 1063
Bethesda, MD 20892-1063
Tel: 301 435 7659
Email: davisl@ninds.nih.gov

or

Patient Recruitment and Public Liaison Office toll-free at:
1-800-411-1222
TTY: 1-866-411-1010

7- The Kessler Foundation in New Jersey –
www.kesslerfoundation.org has some stroke-related research.
Depending on your geography and medical status this could be
helpful. As with the other sites mentioned one could conduct
searches in the cardiology and neurology fields.

8-The Internet Stroke Center – www.strokecenter.org is an
independent web resource for information relating to stroke care
and stroke research. This is a very comprehensive site that is
funded by NIH and NINDS. The Center has a broad Clinical Trial
Registry that you can access by your zip code, and then entering a
mileage range from several pre-selected choices.

Once on the site go to Trial Registry and then a box on the right –
"Search for a Clinical Trials near You". Then put in your zip code
and click on "Locate Clinical Trials". Then you can click on
various mileage points to find the trials. A map comes up and you
will want to look at the column "Status". The studies with a little
**blue head shot are recruiting.**

Click on a study that is recruiting and another screen comes up
with information on study description, eligibility, locations and
contacts and references. I clicked on several studies and got

information which I found to be a bit technical, particularly the descriptions. However, you could take advantage of the contact information and call with questions.

Another suggestion if you or your caregiver is feeling insecure or out of your depth is to make an appointment with your Doctor to get their advice. Go armed with specific questions. You will want to be sure that the study is focusing on a deficit of yours. It's fair to say that working with this site could take some time and effort for the non-clinical person; however the effort could be very worthwhile.

In addition to the information regarding trials the site has a huge amount of information about all aspects of stroke. There are sections with information and resources for patients, families and professionals.

9- ClinLife – www.clinlife.com is a global clinical research website. Started in Europe, it has launched in the US, Canada, and Asia. Its aim is to improve the premises for the conduct of clinical trials and to speed up the development of new, safer medications. They are particularly focused on the speed at which studies get done.

I agree with that focus, as I have observed from my experiences – to my mind there are many ways to speed the clinical research process without hurting results.

The ClinLife home page has a clinical research search engine. You enter the malady, stroke for example, and your zip code and you get results instantly. The web site also has information regarding the clinical research process and other interesting material. The patient can register with the site for email notifications of studies and a newsletter.

**It is important to note that all of these sites are being constantly updated for new studies so it is best to check back on a regular basis for new study opportunities. And as a note, the site**

navigation that I used and described may have changed in the interim between research and today. (I apologize if that happened!)

## Don't just wait for the Alerts.

Getting away from the databases, one might want to investigate the opportunities at more local Hospitals and Hospitals associated with Medical Schools, particularly if they are reasonably convenient to your home. As mentioned in an earlier chapter, these institutions are an excellent place to look for research studies in need of subjects.

Since they conduct many exploratory studies there is an excellent chance that their studies will not be included in the databases. One never can be sure! For example, I doubt the locomotion study in Gainesville would have been in a database since the researcher hadn't yet defined it due to its very exploratory nature. I was the first "guinea pig."

*I get surprised in Naples!*

One day I was sitting in my internist's office at Physicians Regional Hospital in Naples and I noticed posters seeking subjects for several studies being conducted at their clinic, which is what they call their physicians office wing. As it happened, none were for stroke, but it opened my eyes to the possibility that they conduct research. I didn't know that.

And again, that type of research could easily fly underneath the radar of the databases. Now I look around more carefully rather than just reading my magazines and newspapers.

**NOTE: By the way when going to a physician office or hospital, I always bring my own reading material. I think that's a way to prevent the spread of infection to me. Call me paranoid!**

# CHAPTER 27
# ROLE PLAYING DOING CLINICAL RESEARCH

## I Show You What it's like to Participate

*What's it like when you are trying to get into a study or have been accepted?*

In my effort to demystify the clinical research process, I'll describe the various steps I took to get into and then participate in the Boca Raton Spasticity study.

After obtaining information about the study and the contact information from Cure Launcher, I called the administrator to discuss it. She and I chatted about me and the study. Preliminarily, it seemed a good match so the administrator then invited me to their offices to be formally screened against study criteria.

**If I was using one of the databases without the services of the intermediary, Cure Launcher (which is no longer active), I would have utilized the contact information to contact each of the testing locations myself and held a similar conversation.**

Before the first visit to Boca, I assembled my medical records, which can actually take a bit of time. I also made a list of any known allergies, food or otherwise.

Then I sat down and prepared a list of all of the medications that I take, prescription and non-prescription, including any herbs or vitamin supplements. Included on the list was:

The medication by name;
Dosage;
Number of times per day that I take the medication or herb;

When, I started taking it;
And the reason for the substance.

**Incidentally, now that I have completed this list I have it for all of my normal physician visits.** Every time I go to a new doctor, and even at some regular visits, a nurse either asks about my medications or there is redundant paperwork to be completed. It's a drag to have to constantly write them all down.

*Now I just whip out my list.*

I have noticed that the staff is often impressed by my thoroughness and it seems to me that I am taken more seriously. Maybe I am kidding myself.

With respect to clinical research, depending on the exact situation I may be requested to send that information ahead of my first visit. In other cases I just bring it with me, as I did with Boca. In the latter case, the staff copies the information and I am able to keep my original copy.

The first visit was a screening visit. Applying for the spasticity study in Boca Raton, I was greeted in a friendly manner after only a few minutes' wait. Then a nurse interviewed me extensively, explaining the study and its mechanics including any commitments that I had to make.

I would be paid $125.00 per visit to compensate for travel expenses.

The study was in two parts. In the first part there was a possibility of getting a placebo. If I get a placebo then I am not getting any of the medication and I have unluckily been placed in the control group. In this particular study, however, in the second part of the study, which was called an extension study, I was assured of getting the benefit of the chemical injectable being tested.

*I liked that aspect.*

We jointly went over a detailed disclosure document that is called an "informed consent" which I ultimately initialed, signed and received a copy of. It was explained that my privacy was protected as I was only to be known to the sponsor by my initials and a coding system.

The nurse reviewed my medical history, allergy and medication list. That took some time. My blood pressure was taken and an EKG performed.

Next a physical therapist took several detailed measurements of my leg and ankle to see if I met the screening criteria. I did. To establish a benchmark, the therapist timed my walking with and without shoes.

Next, I met with the research neurologist so that she could observe me, review my records and write her observations and notes. It was a friendly conversation. She reviewed the study with me once again.

*I was at the office for several hours. Be prepared.*

I soon learned that I met the criteria, subject to satisfactory blood work and a urine test. An appointment was made for seven days hence and I was told that the second visit would probably be five or six hours in length. They mentioned bringing something to read since there would be some wait times. I was to receive injections in several locations on my leg and thigh.

The urine test was a fasting test so the appointment was at 10 a.m. The nurse suggested that I bring something for breakfast after I gave the urine. Frankly, they should have provided some breakfast. Call me a pain!

During the second visit I completed several questionnaires regarding limb pain and functionality. The physical therapist again measured my leg and I was asked if any of the medications had changed during the intervening week.

After the team reassured themselves that I met the criteria they had to communicate with the sponsor to "randomize" me. This was how they determined which group I was to be in, the full dosage, the half, or the placebo group. In that process they assigned a code and put me in their system.

I knew that I would not be given that information. Since the study was what is called a "blind study" the testing center had no control or knowledge as to which of the three groups I was to be assigned to either.

Once I was randomized the neurologist came in and spent some time determining exactly where I was going to be injected. After being injected, I had to wait about 30 minutes to be sure there were no unexpected side effects. There were none. I was at the office for the expected six hours with no surprises.

An appointment was made for seven days later so that the physical therapist could once again measure my leg at various angles and time my walking. Also, they wanted to determine if there were any unexpected issues. That was a 90 minute appointment. Before leaving that visit I again met with the neurologist to review my progress. An appointment was made for three weeks hence.

That next appointment was also relatively short, again, about 90 minutes. They timed my walking down the hallway again, with and without shoes. The physical therapist measured my leg several ways to see if there were any changes. The nurse and neurologist briefly spoke with me, examined me, and performed a few diagnostic tests. I completed a short questionnaire. My next appointment was to be in about two months.

My fifth visit was a two-hour visit because I was not going to get injected at this time. Originally this was planned to be a transitional visit between the first phase and second extension phase when I would have been injected.

However because of my fall and resulting arm injury my surgeon did not want any other activities except the physical rehabilitation I was undergoing. Bad luck but I could not argue with this. The researcher was to try and get an extension, or at a later date I would get injected through their clinic.

During the two-hour session the researcher took blood, measured my leg, including angles and once again timed my walking with and without shoes. The neurologist chatted with me about progress and reviewed all of the data that had been collected that morning. I also completed two short questionnaires regarding my current health and feelings.

It was confirmed that I would be receiving my travel reimbursements in a few weeks since the first phase was now complete. A few weeks later I received a check for my travel expenses.

# CHAPTER 28
# A STRATEGY FOR THE NEWBIE PARTICIPANT

## Increase the Likelihood of Achieving Success with Clinical Research

The exploratory and approval process for new treatments is long, arduous and complex. Most prospective treatments, pharmaceuticals, medical equipment and techniques wash out sometime during this multi-phase process. Data may show that current techniques are the same or better. Or safety, dosage or cost issues emerge during the research. **Bottom-line, the study results just have not confirmed the earlier expectations.** If you follow the business presses there are numerous announcements from the various pharmaceutical and biotech companies of these failures. These are not happy announcements as the dollars and stakes are often high, particularly when they occur at later phases.

The FDA approval process entails four broad phases requiring human participation on the way to the ultimate approval. In the Phase I trials researchers are trying to confirm their laboratory theories. Studies typically are implemented on a fairly small scale and sometimes with healthy subjects.

At the Phase II stage, the researchers are seeking initial confirmation of disease type treatment success, and initial dosage and side effect data, among other things. These trials are larger than the earlier Phase I studies, but still relatively small.

At the Phase III stage, the trials get substantially larger, into the hundreds or more. Additional confirmations are sorted. There is more information collected on side effects and treatment dosages. For example, the study that I was participating in was a Phase III dosage study. There were about 350 subjects participating in this study, which was being administered by neurological practices around the nation.

At the Phase IV stage the drug or procedure has been approved, however the FDA is tracking the safety, risks and benefits. Also work is still underway to determine the optimal utilization.

There is a prudent strategy particularly for the uninitiated participant who, at once, wants to participate but also wishes to increase their likelihood of successful treatment. **One could limit their participation to studies in phases three and four of the approval process.**

While there are certainly no guarantees, the chance of being treated successfully increases at each phase. In the spirit of "eyes open," however, one could still end up in the placebo group so a prospective participant should carefully understand the study parameters and be willing to live with them. I did.

A second reason to participate in the later stages is that there has been more human testing conducted ahead of you. That's comforting. Still, no guarantee! Developing new things is difficult.

*Personally I have always been willing to assist at any stage of development after I understood the science. But that's me!*

# Part VI

# *Knowledge Is Power*

Remarkable progress is possible when
you know the unknown.

*-Bob Mandell*

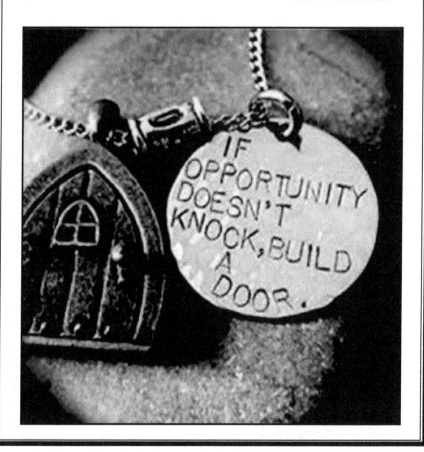

# CHAPTER 29

# A TRANSFORMATIVE MOMENT — BRAIN CHANGE

*Over the 19 years since my stroke I have often hit plateaus. To me, plateau is another word for "brick wall." How to blow the wall down, now, that's the trick! Sometimes I huff, and I puff and I huff some more, and....*

Today, when I think huff and puff to blow the wall down, I think of turning to nontraditional, innovative and integrative approaches. I've done the traditional things, initially made progress and then peaked on many occasions! That's quite typical.

When I think of out-of-the-box, innovative approaches and practitioners who are thought leaders in the area of integrative approaches, I think first of physical therapist, Irene Hujsa, Magic Lady, as I kiddingly call her. Chinese by birth, she grew up in the Philippines and today, with four children, she is married to a successful lawyer. She comes up with innovative therapies that no traditional therapist ever mentioned or suggested. Ever! Part of her magic is having the inquisitive mind to try "the different."

When I started with Irene, I still could not speak publicly. I could not stand up at a networking function and properly introduce myself and my business when the microphone was passed. I just could not do it, and on the rare occasions I tried, the result was pathetic. Yes, I could certainly speak individually, but not the way I speak today. I just didn't have the fluency or the vocabulary.

*So what's the most dramatic thing she has done? And what's the technology?*

That has to be a technique called ETPS which stands for Electro Therapeutic Point Stimulation. This is a hybrid modality used in the treatment of chronic soft tissue pain. Simply, it is low-level micro-current stimulation of acupuncture points. Instead of needling, Irene uses this little micro-current machine to stimulate the points.

Irene has used ETPS on my neck, back, shoulder, and ankle, among other places, primarily to reduce pain and increase functionality. When she is performing ETPS on me, and if it doesn't hurt, I tell her so. Then she goes a little to the right or left or up or down to find the key spot. If it doesn't hurt, then she has not found the key spot. From experience, that's important.

"Does that hurt, how about here," Irene asks

Responding, "No, no, a little bit, that's it!" "Buzz!"

This is a perfect case of "the devil is in the details." It probably sounds sadistic but it works. So I let her do it.

Going back seven or eight years, when Irene first started using this therapy, she was early in her ETPS learning curve. She was curious and since she had seen reduced pain with the initial points she was treating, she suggested hitting my brain. I was leery.

*But I trusted Irene.* In retrospect, a bit scary, maybe, a lot scary, since we didn't actually know what might happen!

*Are you crazy?* Was others' reactions! Some just laughed.

But, I agreed to be treated on my brain. To be specific, the area around the bawi which is the soft spot that everyone has on the top of their heads. Mine is easy to find. (If you didn't take notice of my picture, look on the cover and you'll see why.) So we tried it, slowly and cautiously at first.

*You are dealing with the mysterious brain.*

Coincidentally, I was to receive a Patient of the Year rehabilitation award a few weeks later from a local hospital, NCH, and was scheduled to speak at the Awards ceremony to a group of physicians, therapists and patients. I was nervous and scared. I appreciated the award but not the pressure to speak. So I decided that I would just say thank you to Irene and a few other people and maybe say just a few more sentences. I wouldn't do the Academy Awards "thank you thing." Even if I wanted to I wouldn't have been able to get it out.

Irene treated me two or three times a week for a minute, maybe two. She just worked it into the more traditional therapy she was doing at the time since she was employed by a traditional provider. Initially nothing remarkable was happening, but I've learned that it's a mistake to be too impatient.

One day the week before the Awards Ceremony, suddenly, after Irene treated me, I felt different.

*"I feel different. I can speak publicly. I can speak publicly again!"*

*Unbelievable, this is amazing!* **An Aha moment, if there ever was one!**

When I saw Debbie, I said, *"I can speak publicly again."*
*"What?"* she responded!

*I could just feel it.* Something was substantially different. I just felt it.

*It's hard to describe, it almost seemed that a light went on in my head.* Maybe it did.

So, the day of the awards ceremony, I spoke longer than I had planned and in a reasonable manner. Heck, it was the first time out of the gate. For me, this was a home run. No, this was a grand slam in the seventh game of the World Series.

Ultimately, I bought my own machine to treat myself a minute or so a day. And now, I even travel with it. Initially I was worried about airport security, but we just bury it in our checked luggage. There's nothing lethal about it.

*I don't want to be fuzzy when I am traveling. And when I don't use the machine for a few days, I am.*

People ask curiously what it feels like or if it hurts. Sometimes, when the machine is on, I can feel my brain almost rattling, and a dizzy feeling, but it passes. And it doesn't really hurt. If for some reason I don't do my ETPS for a few days, I can tell the difference. I'm not as sharp.

Not only did my speech improve, but, amazingly, my creative juices all of a sudden exploded.

The week of my big Aha moment, I woke up every night and went into the bathroom where I could put the light on without disturbing Debbie, to write down some project notes, so as not to forget my thoughts.

*Sometimes, I have the greatest ideas at night and I better write them down, otherwise I might forget.*

**It all started one week. What a week. God had to be watching, and I hope, cheering!**

READER NOTE: More recently ETPS was renamed MPS for Micro-current Point Stimulation Therapy (mpstherapy.com). If a reader were looking on the internet for this therapy they might want to use the more current name in addition to the older name.

SECOND READER NOTE: The Avazzia therapy that will be discussed in Chapter 33 of the book accomplishes the same thing with no pain and I will be getting one of their machines in the future. These days when I see Irene she uses the newer Avazzia machine which has a feedback mechanism which helps her to determine the point location without the discomfort.

# CHAPTER 30

# DISAPPOINTMENT WITH TRADITIONAL ACUPUNCTURE

*I have been surprised, but not in a good way!*

Since the stroke I have tried acupuncture on several occasions with very mixed results. My most successful experience was early during my recovery, actually at Mediplex. I found out that one of the staff physical therapists was also a trained acupuncturist and she wanted to treat me.

Likewise, Debbie and I were anxious to try anything as I worked to recover. Initially, the administrators at the Mediplex nursing home resisted using their facility for private treatments because of insurance and liability considerations. An accommodation was made to allow the therapist to treat me in her off-hours, since at the time I was not allowed to leave the nursing home except for emergencies or physician visits.

Since the treatments were late in the day, Debbie attended. She always said that the therapist put her whole energy and soul into those needles. And I did feel better from those few treatments. Unfortunately, after a few sessions the therapist announced that she was leaving the nursing home, and Connecticut, to return to Alaska for family reasons. That ended that.

After leaving the nursing home and heading home to Ridgefield about six weeks later, we found an Asian gentleman who also performed acupuncture in Wilton, Connecticut which is not too far from Ridgefield.

*Nothing is happening. This is just a rip off!*

After a few unremarkable sessions, I stopped. Debbie thought he was just in it for the money. He also sold us some Chinese herbs, dried roots and things, which were not only disgusting to the taste, but also seemingly accomplished nothing. Were they preserved properly? It didn't look like it, but maybe we were wrong. It was a blind item for us. Nothing constructive seemed to happen from any of it. Rightly or wrongly that experience turned us off to acupuncture for years.

I recently read a case study that Dr. Charles Shang prepared in 2005, that showed progress using acupuncture and herbs together. My gut says that this should be helpful, even if it wasn't for me. But I think it's highly dependent on the practitioner knowing their points and having good quality herbs and the correct herbal formula.

Thirteen or fourteen years later we were on an Oceania cruise ship in which Canyon Ranch ran the spa services. They were offering discounts on the acupuncture, so I tried three sessions with a gentleman acupuncturist and later added a fourth since it was working. My neck pain remarkably disappeared and I was so excited. I even tried to plot a way to meet up with him on another cruise but we lost contact. He did know his points.

*Frustration!*

Unfortunately, after a few weeks, the pain returned. Perhaps I was expecting too much. Maybe my stroke and other medical issues were too complex for the technique since they occurred so long ago.

Others have had better results than I with acupuncture. **But what I have learned is that unless the practitioner really knows their points well, these treatments are a waste of time and money.** That's the same with the ETPS treatments that I had so much success with and discussed in Chapter 29.

What I hypothesize with stroke, is that the electrical stimulation on the acupuncture points, gives the extra "jolt" (no pun intended) that makes the difference for my long-standing issues.

A question one might ask, how do I know if an acupuncturist or a therapist in any of these alternative therapies is competent since it is so important?

Initially, I look at their backgrounds, but it's not easy because I am less familiar with the schools, so I am practical and results oriented.

*If I don't feel a difference, I stop. If I feel short-term improvements I give it a bit of time, perhaps a month. But if it keeps fading, I stop out of frustration.*

While I have had little long term benefits from traditional acupuncture, I presume others have had far more constructive outcomes. And for those who had more positive results, I say – great, keep at it. Everyone is different and their issues are certainly also different!

And I realize that there are those who will continue even if they only get short-term pain relief, and that's obviously a personal decision. Chronic pain is no fun. *Good luck*

# CHAPTER 31

# A LITTLE KNOWN THERAPY THAT WORKED

Through Irene, I have been exposed to a series of innovative therapies in addition to the ETPS. Many of these therapies are not well known, even by professional therapists. I find this a bit remarkable; however these therapies have been an important part of my recovery. Let me tell you about a few.

**The MyoKinesthetic System -** (www.myokinesthetic.com/)

One day during the spring of 2013, Irene called me out of the blue,

"Bob, I have something new that I think might help you, want to try it? Just half hour sessions; it's called MYK." She had attended weekend training on the therapy with Dr. Mike Uriarte, a chiropractor from Overland Park, Kansas, who was the founder.

I was hopeful, but very skeptical that at this stage in the game anything could really make a difference. But, I've also learned that it is best to give anything new in therapy a 30-day try. Then if it's not working, go on to something else or just stop. A little patience is needed.

*Still with Irene, you never know. She is always coming up with something new, and often, whatever it is, works.*

I decided to go for it. So just what is this new technique that she had learned?

MYK is a non-invasive muscle movement technique that corrects and balances the nervous system. The system is used in connection with painful or limited range of motion issues like I have on my entire right side. Also, the technique is used for nerve and muscle pain in connection with many diseases unrelated to stroke.

From a lay perspective, the technique combines muscle stimulation with the identification of specific nerve endings. It is a neurological augmentation to massage therapy. The innovative technique treats all of the muscles along one particular nerve pathway. Irene massages one muscle at a time – now that's different!

The plan was that Irene would begin treating my leg to see if my gait would improve, and if it did, she would start to treat my shoulder and arm. In a 30-minute session there was only time for one area to be treated properly.

There was no change during the first few visits but Irene encouraged me to give it some time. During the second or third week, we started to see a dramatic change. I walked around Irene's office at the end of a session and there definitely was a difference, both with respect to speed and gait. Irene was excited, I was ecstatic, but still skeptical. Trying new techniques, often I have experienced improvements during a session only to see them fade away. Frustrating!

"Let's see if it sticks," I often say to Irene.

But it was sticking. My walking was improving a remarkable amount, and I was super excited. At home, I could now walk around our tile floor without shoes or socks. That was a first. Also, my ankle seemed to be strengthening allowing me to walk on more varied outdoor surfaces like grass and sand.

*I was sooo excited by the results.*

How to find this therapy? As part of his practice, Dr. Uriarte runs weekend training sessions in MYK. His website, shown above has a search engine where certified therapists are listed by geography. Depending on the geography there are various numbers of certified therapists listed. In Florida, there are quite a number, up north less so.

# CHAPTER 32

# A SUDDEN DETOUR FROM REHABILITATION

*Like a bolt of lightning – she hits - and down on my back I go!*

One Friday evening, late June 2013, we were exiting from a pleasant enough dinner with a friend of Debbie's in our former country club's tavern. Then the unexpected occurred. Debbie was walking her friend out towards the front entrance, and they had stopped to chat for a minute.

Suddenly her friend looked up at me, and screams out that she has to say good-bye, which she had already done. She then bolts towards me as if I was getting off a plane returning from Iraq. As she was running, her sandals caught in the carpet turning her into an airborne missile. She slammed into me, knocking me down on my back.

Running over, Debbie said that I turned white, and she was fearful that I was going to pass out or worse - have some kind of attack. Guests and the club staff had quickly gathered over me as I rolled around, trying to assess my condition saying, "give me a minute - give me a minute." I was trying to get into a more comfortable position. The woman was screaming apologizes.

*It hurts – damn it! She has jeopardized my health!*

I was still hurting over the weekend and was unable to get out of bed without Debbie pulling me up. It hurt like heck as I sat up. Something was wrong!

Early Monday morning, before breakfast I was still in pain, after taking pain killers. I decided to drive the mile or so over to the hospital to try and sort this out.

We have learned, as with Caryn and her therapists, mentioned in Chapter 19, that it is important to find out where the physicians I am planning to see have been trained. So, before I see someone, I research their medical training. That tells me at least two very important things – are they bright and have they been trained by a well-known and rigorous school.

In today's global economy, I sometimes encounter medical professionals from foreign countries. There are many offshore schools that have equally high standards worthy of consideration. When this occurs I take some extra time to do my medical due diligence, looking at the school faculty, where the staff has trained, where medical personnel have licenses and where they have practiced. With regard to physicians I look for Board certifications and honors. My one caveat is that since I only speak English, they must be fluent in my language to prevent any miscommunications.

Usually, I check on the internet for the prospective physician's background before making an appointment. There are sites on the internet where you may find patient reviews and where any negative information may be mentioned. In addition when I go to a physician's office I start looking for diplomas, board certifications, awards – whatever is on the wall. I always read these certificates, and if I don't see anything, then I politely ask what schools the doctor has gone to.

Also, sometimes, when initially chatting with the doctor, I have been known to ask how their grades were. That usually gets a chuckle! But based on my experience, the conversation becomes more constructive and we are taken much more seriously with more physician face-time when I do my "little college bit." I can see it in their eyes and how they appraise me.

*Sometimes they even ask if I am a physician.*

The orthopedic surgeon who I had my visit with had graduated from Columbia and U of Michigan Medical School. Great! - Upon reading the MRI he concluded that I had two fractured vertebrae on my spine.

Surgery was scheduled for three days hence. They performed a 21$^{st}$ Century technique he carefully explained to me, called Kyphon Balloon Kyphoplasty. In this technique the surgeon inserts a balloon in each of the vertebrae breaks and fills them with cement. It's done as an outpatient procedure with light anesthesia. And I was finished and headed home before noon that very morning of the surgery, though, with additional pain killers.

Next, I had to deal with ankle pain from the incident. Debbie said that she saw my ankle turn as I went down. X-rays and an MRI! The podiatrist thought I might have a hairline fracture and suggested a boot. That would mean that my walking would be more challenged and possibly unsafe with the balance issues so I opted to see if Irene could assist with her therapies.

*The experimental MYK therapy I was successfully doing with Irene was out, and for the time being, no daily physical fitness! Not Good! - What a disaster that this progress had to stop!*

This was a disheartening experience. No question! Honestly, I felt a victim rather than a victor. Friends said to me, "You were doing so well and now this!" And it took some time to shake that attitude.

Look, I'm human too. But, I couldn't undo it, and with the pain, I couldn't ignore it.

What's the saying, *"Pick yourself up, dust yourself off and start all over again!"*

# CHAPTER 33

# GETTING BACK ON TRACK WITH MORE INNOVATIVE THERAPIES

In July 2013, after being tackled, physically, I wasn't able to get back to MYK. I had to deal with my broken back, balance issues emanating from the fall and an injured ankle. Recovering from the back surgery, I was disgusted with my condition. All that time and money improving with MYK was out the window! My daily workouts had stopped and I was spending hours in doctor's waiting rooms and offices. I was at Physician's Regional so much that people greeted me by name as I walked around.

Traditional therapy had been prescribed, which I started. I also decided to talk with Irene about what supplement and possibly innovative techniques she might have up her sleeve. I wanted to get on top of this fast having smelt a whiff of big change. Additionally, her take on the more traditional would hopefully speed up my recovery as she often used techniques which were a bit different.

*"Irene, help, help!"*

*"Irene, what do you suggest?"* Leave it to her…

*"Horse Therapy"* she responded. *"What, you've got to be kidding?"*

**Horse Therapy** (www.pemf.com)

Yep, that's right. Horse Therapy!

Am I a horse! Nah, Nah! *"Come on Irene."*

As much as I trust Irene, this sounded like too much, even for me. I had to laugh. Still, this is Irene talking. She quickly produced a sales brochure in which there were testimonials from NFL players attesting to its worthiness. I was stunned.

Horse therapy speeds the healing of bone injuries in racing horses. It has been used extensively at Churchill Downs and many other racing venues. Most importantly she said, "The same technique that works on a horse also turns out to work on a human." Remember, at our core, we are all animals.

*Hard to believe*

Irene explained that the scientific name for Horse Therapy is Pulsed Electromagnetic Field (PEMF). It's a non-invasive technique that uses this little machine which emits a full spectrum of frequencies to retune cellular signaling in the body. This in turn heals the bone injuries. Additionally, PEMF is used for arthritis, inflammation, pain reduction and boosts to the immune system.

"Here, look at this little machine. Watch what happens when I turn it on. I am going to tape it to your back." The lights went on in a pattern but there was nothing to feel.

*How is this going to fix my back, I thought?*

In a few treatments I was feeling a difference. Irene loaned me a machine. Debbie taped it to my back, and ankle in the injured spots, and kept it on for about 45 minutes in each location. Truly unbelievable!

A few weeks later, Irene starts telling me about a new model she was waiting for. This one is called a Full Spectrum Magnetic Field Generator, and the difference is that an additional set of frequencies has been added. She said that this one would work even better.

Not only has it worked, but the machine has other applications. For example, it makes stomach aches go away and Irene says wrinkles also.

*"Come on! I cracked?"*

Amazingly, it does help with the stomach. When Debbie gets a stomach ache, as she is prone to, she puts it over her navel for about a half an hour and the discomfort disappears. Do you believe it! We are still working on the wrinkle bit. And there are lots of other uses we are just exploring.

An anecdote. Just recently we were at an education session for some new dermatological procedures that Debbie was interested in. The speaker said the technology was PEMF. He was asking if anyone in the audience had heard of it. My hand shot up, the speaker was shocked someone knew. I spoke with him for a few minutes mentioning that we had a machine, a portable one. Not like the one he was showing, which was much larger, but the same technology. Debbie just shook her head, saying "I can't believe you knew this, and we have a machine." I said, *"Irene said it worked on wrinkles."*

So where to research, perhaps you can Google some of the key words in this write-up. The portable machines are available from several vendors. Demonstrations in selected dermatological offices are ongoing, for the larger equipment. My focus remains my back.

There's more....

**COLD LIGHT LASER** (www.spine-health.com)

For several years, Irene had been pitching a technique using a cold laser machine. It never did anything for me and she came to realize it was probably just not strong enough. But more recently she told me about newer laser equipment that she had ordered. She was very excited that it would help me.

The newer equipment arrived. It is a hand-held device that is 20 times more intense than her previous equipment. Not only does it emit a stronger energy, but the beam is more focused and concentrated, a dual advantage.

This therapy, which is called Cold Light Laser, utilizes light to stimulate cell types such as muscles, ligaments and nerves. Irene's recent purchase looks a bit like a flash light however; in this case non-thermal photons of light are emitted. Unlike the earlier equipment, this stronger energy model was definitely working.

Cold Light Laser can also be used for more maladies than just stroke therapy. Positive results have been observed for back, neck and knee pain emanating from causes such as arthritis, tendonitis, fibromyalgia and carpal tunnel syndrome.

It also turns out that the newer, more concentrated, and incidentally pain-free model can be substituted for the painful ETPS machine. It seems like the gain is there, and the pain of the ETPS machine is gone, a significant leap forward.

But I still think the model that hurts is better at finding the key points.

Anyway, Irene places the beam on my acupuncture points, including my scalp Bawi, just like she did with the ETPS machine. I still sort of vaguely wonder about putting this strong laser on my head, but we do it. And nothing bad has happened, only good!

## ESSENTIAL OILS (www.doterra.com/us/)

*Now it's time to get soothing!*

During the past year or two, Irene has introduced doTerra essential oils into her practice, integrating them into her treatments. She had been to some corporate training and became convinced that these oils were a leap forward. This manufacturer appears very scientifically and naturally based. In many cases the oils are quite soothing, and others, seem to provide a surprising level of relief for particular problems.

My initial reaction to the oils having never experienced them was that they were a bit of "black magic." But they felt good when she massaged them into my ankle, back, neck and shoulder. So what's so bad! But I was amazed by one of the oils, marjoram. Absolutely shocked!

I'll tell you. Since I had my stroke, there has been a substantial increase in right side cramping, from the tips of my toes, to my shoulder, arm, and everything in between. My circulation is still constrained and I assume that this is at least part of the reason for the cramping as I rarely experience it on my non-effected side.

Up until recently the best answer was consuming a lot of water, though I still cramped. And I've tried other remedies with little success. The typical scenario is that I have a leg cramp, which then spreads up my right side, typically occurring during the night, while in bed. When I cramp my spasticity increases. And if you also suffer from cramping, you know that cramps hurt like heck.

Irene suggested using marjoram. The oil is amazing! Marjoram stops the cramps in their tracks. When I get a leg cramp, Debbie rubs marjoram into the bottoms of my feet. Almost miraculously, within a minute or two at the most, the cramps disappear. They stay away for several days. Marjoram helps Debbie also. When she gets a severe leg cramp, as she often does, and she gets some duzzies, this oil knocks them out in a minute or two. The downside, they do smell, in some cases not wonderfully, but by adding the Peppermint oil the odor is greatly reduced.

I also use some of the other oils, Deep Blue and Wintergreen for neck and muscle pain and On Guard to ward off sickness that one catches when flying. I usually use the On Guard capsules.

Recently, I gave some Peppermint oil to a friend who had been suffering with migraine headaches for years. I also explained to her how to utilize the oil. When I saw her the next morning she was all smiles – the oil had miraculously worked. Then her boyfriend wanted some oil also for his issues.

One cautionary note, these oils can be a bit pricey. To us, they are well worth the cost, but that's a personal decision. Pain relief without ingesting medication is certainly a big plus!

## AVAZZIA THERAPY

*This is amazing! The march of technology results in remarkable progress!*

In mid-October 2014 Irene spoke to me about a new device she had received from First Alternatives (www.firstalternativetherapies.com). One of her good friends suggested using it to see if she could confirm the remarkable results her friend was getting. Irene couldn't wait to see if it would help with my treatments.

Describing it to me, Irene mentioned that she had started using the device as a replacement for the ETPS which tended to be more painful during therapy. All excited about it, she suggested that it might help to improve my walking and balance which still were, and are an issue since the falls.

Naturally, I readily agreed to be treated! She began running the relatively small electrical stimulator up and down my spine, starting at the base. She explained that these devices use micro-current to target the c-fibers of the nervous system, stimulating neuropeptides and other regulatory peptides that the body uses to heal itself.

The way it works is that she receives a starting number in a particular spot, and then, as she treats my back, for example, the number decreases if progress is being made. If the number is "sticky", then she must spend extra time on the particular spot to get the desired effect. Regarding my feeling the electrical stimulator, on several occasions she adjusted the stimulation to reduce any potential therapy discomfort as treatment is not supposed to be painful. As I was being treated I thought, "Well, this is quite magical!"

Tim Smith, who spent decades with Texas Instruments, invented this technology. He has an impressive record of success having developed the first computer chips for the Apple and IBM PC, and played an instrumental role on the Apollo Lunar Modules.

To quote Mr. Smith, "I've been an inventor and design engineer all my life. I retired from TI but my brain didn't retire. I met someone who was being treated for foot pain because of diabetes and who was worried about amputation. I could immediately see in my brain how to design a product to make treatment better and more effective."

At this writing I have had eleven treatments and can see dramatic improvements with my walking with some pain reduction in my neck, back and shoulder. Since we started on my spine my uppers have only been treated twice. I think that I already feel some improved range of motion. We'll have to monitor progress but I am extremely enthusiastic about my initial results.

If you are looking for a practitioner in your geography I suggest you email info@firstalternativetherapies.com or call (954) 554-4897 and they will put you in touch with a trained medical professional.

**I spoke with Michael Legal, CEO of the company, and he was so moved by my story that he wanted to assist my community. He offered $100 off any Avazzia purchase if you mention this book or type in the promo code "victor" on the website. This will assist me to help other stroke survivors.**

Irene has been so impressed with the results she has been getting with the Avazzia Equipment and Therapy that she will be conducting training sessions for First Alternatives to spread the word.

## EASTERN BASED THERAPIES

I've previously described waking up after the stroke with a loss of feeling on my entire right side. And, unfortunately, along with the feeling, went my blood flow. If I get a cut on my right side, it takes much longer to heal because the blood flows much more slowly than on my unaffected side. For that reason, Irene has focused on therapies to increase my blood flow.

That's where Far Eastern based approaches come in.

## GUA SHA (www.guasha.cm)

The first of these modalities is Gua Sha, which Irene has utilized on my back, neck, and down my right side. This is a traditional Chinese technique considered to be in the acupuncture family. In recent years it has gained adherents in the West, as more research shows positive indications.

Gua Sha is used for pain relief, both chronic and acute. In addition, Gua Sha can also be a therapeutic approach to achieve anti-inflammatory effects. The technique increases blood flow to the areas being treated. Exactly what I need! After Irene massages oil into my skin she literally scrapes the skin with a little straight-edged implement. The idea is to scrape away the restrictions. It has helped increase my right-sided feeling, a bit, though it is still much challenged. She also uses Gua Sha to reduce my neck pain.

Gua Sha is not only a stroke technique, but is used for many other conditions like muscle spasms and fibrotic tissue chronic pain. One thing to note, and it isn't good: Gua Sha can leave some pretty nasty skin marks and soreness. When Debbie first saw them, she was shocked. "What happened to you?" They do, however, normally disappear in a few days.

## CUPPING (www.cuppingtherapy.org)

Another Eastern approach that Irene uses to increase blood flow is cupping. Once again, this therapy has its roots in ancient history. Irene puts these suction cups on my back, which seems to mobilize the blood flow. The suction effect can be adjusted. When the cup does its job it automatically releases from the skin, which I know sounds kind of weird. But it does seem to work. This technique also leaves marks, but is not as uncomfortable as Gua Sha. These techniques can be Googled in your geography to find a practitioner.

These non-traditional integrative approaches that I have described are certainly extraordinarily constructive.

# CHAPTER 34

## BALANCE THERAPY – AURICULOTHERAPY

It was January 2014, and my balance was still challenged from the earlier injury. Unfortunately, I fell in our kitchen and fractured the humerus bone in my right shoulder. A bad break! (Again, no pun intended.) My already challenged balance had now become even more problematic.

*This has not been a good year! This balance issue has to be solved!*

*I have come to realize that if I am out there, you never know where the next opportunity lies! And also, who I am going to meet, who might have a new solution.*

Attending the Imagine Solutions Conference in Naples I described earlier, I met the lovely and sophisticated Dr. Mary Bonnette, who fortunately was sitting at my lunch table. I was telling her about this book over lunch, and the fact that I was having balance issues, affecting my ability to walk safely. She had observed the other kind people at the table assisting me on the grass. During our conversation, Mary quietly said that one of the issues she focused on at her Neurotherapy Center, was balance. She got my interest and I quickly arranged to visit her in Ft. Myers.

The integrative therapy technique Mary utilizes is something called Auriculotherapy (ATENS). First developed by the French neurologist Paul Nogier, it is a form of integrative medicine. It is based on the idea that the ear is a microsystem reflecting the entire brain, which is represented on the auricle, the outer portion of the ear.

Everyone is different, so once again, this is a personalized approach to restoring energetic balance. This is accomplished by removing the underlying blockages that may be causing a disease or condition, like poor balance. This then allows the body to heal itself by redirecting system energy through signaling body molecules, to create neutrality and natural balance of mood, thought and physical symptoms.

Besides balance issues, ATENS has applications in pain reduction, addiction treatment, smoking and stress management, among others. It is a chemical-free, non-invasive treatment approach, which has been shown to also help in general health and wellness programs.

Mary treats me using painless electro-stimulation to the surface of the ear. She uses a Stim Flex machine, which stimulates the ear nerve endings in the relevant points for the particular malady. Other practitioners may use needles which is then referred to as ear acupuncture and also manual stimulation, which is termed ear reflexology.

The Auriculotherapy Certification Institute (ACI) is North America's only organization to offer certification specifically in auriculotherapy, auricular acupuncture, and auricular medicine. In addition, ACI recognizes the contributions to this field, both by ear acupuncture practitioners in China, and by doctors of auricular medicine in Europe. So this is a global integrative medical technique.

Their website (www.auriculotherapy.org) has a search function to find practitioners by geography.

I had my first treatment, which initially left me dizzy, but by the following morning I definitely showed promise of improving my balance. I was quite impressed! My next several treatments resulted in a bit more progress.

*This is working!* During my next several visits I felt that my balance was continuing to improve. Moving forward a month or so…

I have been informally assisting Mary with her new brochure.

"The picture of the brain you have looks scary to me. How about putting a picture of an ear on the front? That's what you are treating to deal with the various maladies." We found a great picture, which at once showed the ear, the various points and the maladies to be treated. *"That's it! Put that on the cover or in the brochure."*

Looking at all of the problems that could be treated, I noticed "muscle tightness." "Let's try this on me today." And we did!

Another good day! The next day I could feel a difference. I'm walking faster and my arm feels looser, after just one treatment of a very few minutes. **Unbelievable!**

*This could be big! I'm continuing to get treatments, and have increased the frequency to twice a week... Still, this is a work in progress... Good Progress!*

# CHAPTER 35

# ADDITIONAL THOUGHTS ON INTEGRATIVE AND INNOVATIVE THERAPIES

*So how would I sum this up?*

Based on my considerable conversations with medical research professionals, clinicians, and lay consumers alike, it seems like very few have heard of these therapies and procedures. When I mention them, people's eyes glass over and they readily admit to not knowing about them. For example, at a recent scientific meeting I attended, no one with whom I spoke had heard of ETPS or MYK. I didn't even go into the other therapies, though I have met a few people who were vaguely familiar with ear acupuncture and, in some cases, the Eastern Medicine approaches.

*Why don't people know about these therapies?*

From my perspective, many factors contribute to this phenomenon including the traditional structure of the US healthcare quagmire, the tradition-based insurance reimbursement system and the nature of traditional medical training and belief.

Furthermore, many of these therapies do not have what I like to term, FDA quality research to back their claims, so of course there will be skepticism among traditionalists.

Also, there has been a general lack of cohesive and effective marketing efforts and advocacy by practitioners of these non-traditional integrative therapies. Hence, little marketing or communication.

Finally and importantly, these therapies are typically not covered by insurance, so the patient must pay on their own. For many, this is either an emotional or financial detriment, or both. The fact that it should not be so, is irrelevant.

**I've tried to briefly describe a world with many little known innovative and integrative therapies. In my opinion, the game-changing approach means entering and embracing this world. That's been my experience.**

**Remember my Chinese dinner story. These therapies are all in Column B and I believe at least some are required if one wants to maximize their recovery. Like my parents said, "at least try it."**

**When I plateau using the traditional, I seek out alternatives rather than accepting the plateau. That's the Victor way. You too!**

*Something to keep in mind, so you are not surprised, or put off!*

Some caveats! One may find skepticism regarding the efficacy of these techniques. I did. My experience has been that this has come from the traditionalists in the healthcare field. Because there has been a general lack of broad training and advocacy by adherents of these techniques, those trained in traditional approaches have not had the necessary exposure. It's unfortunate. These skeptics will often say something like, "there's no research to support the claims" or some such thing. And as I said earlier, they are correct in many cases. While I don't want to take issue with this stance, **I know what has worked for me. And I am delighted. But I also understand where the traditionalists are coming from!**

*Just something else to keep in mind as you or the caregiver delves into non-traditional therapies.*

Unfortunately, the availability of practitioners of each of these approaches is a mixed bag. It seems to be very geography dependent.

There are training courses to teach therapists all of these techniques. But they are far from ubiquitous, and the training seminars are often expensive for the students to attend. As thought-leaders, Irene and Mary participate in some of the training programs but far from all.

Sometimes they play leadership roles, teaching particular modules, or courses, and sometimes, they are students. Recently, Mary ran a workshop at Johns Hopkins University in Baltimore, MD. Irene is constantly being asked to run, or actively participate in various workshops and seminars.

Finally, one additional thought that should be mentioned: while there are other therapists in other geographies who utilize these techniques, they may not use the same integrative approach that, for example, Irene does. Or the same technique, or equipment, that Mary prefers. Of course, these other professionals may also have their own interpretive approaches.

And who is to say who is better for each patient. This is customized medicine and every patient is different. Certainly every stroke patient is different with varied issues and nuances. That's what makes stroke so tough.

*My patient perspective suggests a proactive stance by the patient or caregiver, and also diligence. And then the frustrating need to give these approaches time to make an impact. But it can be, sooo worth it!*

Knowledge is power! If there is a need, a sincere good luck!

*In my Stroke Coaching role---can I assist? Please contact me at bob@strokevictor.com.*

# Part VII

# *Lifestyles After Stroke*

The New Us Succeed.

*- Bob Mandell*

If you want something in your life you've never had,
you'll have to do something,
you've never done.

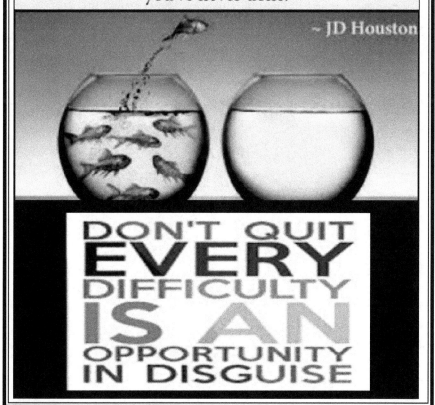

~ JD Houston

DON'T QUIT
EVERY
DIFFICULTY
IS AN
OPPORTUNITY
IN DISGUISE

# CHAPTER 36
# SEX AFTER STROKE

*Don't be shy! Don't be reticent! Focus on what you can do, not what you can't!*

*—Bob and Debbie Mandell*

Intimacy and sex are part of humanity, a very important part. They are basic needs of humans through the ages. Without sex none of us would exist, I would not be writing this book and you would not be reading it. It is in the Bible, as it is in so many other writings.

Then why the skittishness when it comes to talking about sex? Me too! When I started to write this book, I had contemplated covering the subject but will readily admit to being reluctant to go into details. A bit personal and maybe embarrassing, I thought.

One weekend, I was discussing this book with a business coach of mine, David. I handed him my chapter outline, which did not include any chapters on intimacy or sex. He took one look at it and screamed at me as he often does,

*"Where's the sex? You said you were doing a book about hope after stroke. Where's the hope without the intimacy and the sex?"* He then took a phone call that dragged on for a while which gave me time to think.

*"Yes, this is too important a subject to ignore,"* I agreed. He was not talking about treating the subject only clinically. *"It's not motivational if you don't get into it a bit. What's possible if you let yourself go, disability or not?"* he went on. We talked about it and then I said, *"If I am going to do this, I have to get Debbie onboard."*

She was in the next office working. David said, *"Let me talk to her.*

*Get her in here."* He went into a whole explanation and finished by shouting, *"Do you want Bob's book to help people? Do you want the book to sell? He needs to talk about intimacy and sex and how, if you have a disability, you can still have a life."* It's an important message.

Reluctant at first, she finally bought into it. *"If it will help, then let's do it."*

So, with that as an introduction, here goes,

We had been married for only 18 months before the stroke, and then in a nursing home my penis had shriveled. It, like my other plumbing was on vacation as the nurses were accompanying me to the bathroom. Not real pleasant.

So, just how long was the vacation to last or would it ever end, was the sixty-four thousand dollar question. Unfortunately, many stroke survivors stay that way. Clearly, worrisome! But, fortunately, as time went by I no longer needed assistance in the bathroom. However, my other plumbing was another story; I was still not able to get hard. Of course I was embarrassed by my situation. Wouldn't every red-blooded guy be embarrassed? I vowed to do something. At least try.

*I wasn't discussing this. This was a secret between me and me.*

Starting to think…what do I do if my leg hurts? I massage it. If my arm hurts, I rub it to make it feel better. You have the idea! If my hand is numb, I massage it. So I started to massage it, to masturbate. But for several weeks it remained soft, nothing happened. This was getting more worrisome, even in my challenged intellectual state. *I have to get it going again,* I thought!

I also started doing some simple meditation exercises. Deep breathing, relaxing, nothing fancy! I had never done this before.

A few weeks later, *what do we have here?* I smiled to me. It was finally and miraculously showing some life. It was hard, though frankly a long way from what I had been used to pre-stroke.

Next step, I wondered if I would be able to satisfactorily perform when the time came. But that was for another day. Still, clearly progress…a darn good thing.

I can't say if the improving situation was normal body healing that coincidentally occurred, the masturbation, the meditation, plain luck, God having mercy or a combination. I'll never know.

*Who cares, I could get hard! This was a Big Aha Day.*

When Debbie visited that day, I told her the big news. Kissing me, she was obviously happy but acted as though she hadn't thought much about it until that moment. *I think she had other things on her mind.*

*We're off and running!*

Fast forward a bit. No discussion of sex with disabilities can be complete without referencing the pharmaceutical Viagra and its competitors. **And the most important thing I have to say is that one should talk with his doctor about the opportunities, risks and cautions when, and if, they use these medications. I did. And, in addition, as the Viagra advertisement mentions, check with your physician as to advisability of sexual activity.**

Our experience with these pharmaceuticals has been, admittedly, minimal. There was concern with the potential for drug interactions, given the list of things I take. Still, we thought that we might try.

A funny story, though I must say I didn't think so at the time. Several months after I had gotten home my urologist said we should try Viagra and gave me a few samples. So one Saturday afternoon we decided to give it a whirl and I took the little blue pill.

We started getting friendly, as we anxiously waited for it to work.

Suddenly the phone rings and though I said to let it ring, Debbie picked it up. It was her son, Keith, who said he had decided to surprise us and was in Ridgefield five minutes away. Keith had never before surprised us, always making prior arrangements to visit.

What a weird coincidence! Thank God he called giving us a few minutes to literally *"not get caught with our pants down."* Well, that took care of that as we rapidly dressed. But I was feeling dizzy soon after, presumably from the Viagra pill, and so we never tried that again.

For our other experience, mindful of the earlier dizziness with Viagra, I tried the small dosage of Cialis. Unfortunately there was no noticeable positive effect. It's not surprising since the small dosage pill is meant to be taken daily and I have been reluctant to do that. So there is no surprise that there was no positive impact. I would have to acknowledge that we have not given it a fair trial. Maybe we will some time.

Still…

# CHAPTER 37
# LOVING CONNECTIONS

Suffering a stroke or any disability is ugly, let's not kid ourselves. So, for many, the last thing on their mind is sex. Furthermore, after the stroke lots of times my right side hurt. It still does, and it probably always will, at least to some extent. Pull on my-still-partly-paralyzed arm, it hurts. My right leg hurts with every step. None of this is fun. And as many know, therapy also often hurts.

*For a change of pace, wouldn't it be nice to have something pulled or touched that felt good?*

I have spoken with many people in this situation and they are focused on going to doctors, making various arrangements, therapy of one kind or another depending on the survivor's deficits and, in some cases, complicated financial and living issues, among other things. Little or no thought of sex.

These folks, like us, are overwhelmed, regardless of education, profession or financial standing. Just overwhelmed! Where do I turn next? What do I do now?

*So why is this screwball talking about, sex! What's he thinking?*

This book is about hope. Without it, it's too easy for the dragon, the enemy, depression to make its ugly appearance. With depression, we risk a slippery slope downward! And down. And the more down, the harder to get up.

**So even more important than hope, this book is also about doing – making the hope happen!**

So to keep depression at bay…*we have learned that the psyche has to be more positive. And to my mind there is nothing more constructive than intimacy and yes, sex!*

Hope – depression; hope – depression; hope – depression; HOPE AND ACTION!

*Still, in this bleak time, easier said than done! How to start, where to start?*

And, really importantly, we had to consider the fact that I was pretty unsure of myself in the sex department after the stroke. Debbie less so, but she wanted it to be successful. So how to start with performance anxiety as a real underlying concern.

Out of my psychological readings about Masters and Johnson, the sexologists, they developed a non-pressurized go-slow technique which was essentially a One-Step-At-A-Time process.

*Let's go back to the one-step-at-a-Time lesson! That lesson applies to many things, not just walking or physical therapy. There it is, again.*

The way to start then was with some physical contact. I am talking about the entire gestalt of sex, not just the physical. The warmth, the loving camaraderie, the feelings, and yes, at some point the physical!

**Compare these,**

In the nursing home, I'm sitting in my wheel chair. Debbie enters, kisses me deeply and strokes my neck and head. Doesn't that feel good, darn right? Nothing outright sexual here, just warmth and feeling!

*Compared to,*

Debbie enters with a peck on the lips or cheek and then starts talking about one thing or another. Or worse, doesn't even bother with the peck. Every couple is different.

*What feels better for both survivor and caregiver?*

That's a way to start, very simply because part of One-Step-at-a-Time is having small successes, even tiny successes and avoiding big failures, blow-ups.

So, go slow with this,

Moving forward, I am in bed, Debbie sits on the side lowering the bed guards if they are present, and either leans over or climbs in and we just hold each other. Perhaps lightly touch one another, non-sexual touching at the beginning.

*But isn't that sexy?*

*Doesn't that lead too nicer feelings for both? Isn't that different than Debbie just sitting in a chair and talking with me? The talk can come later! Imagine a bit, doesn't that sound better, warmer, more loving?*

*Repeat the successes. Repeat the scene in bed. There was only so much one could do. The action is always a little different anyway.*

*Hope acted out. Slowly and one-step-at-a-time! Be happy, not sad or depressed.*

*Another step, Debbie climbs into bed and there is more feeling, just touching. Both of us! And so on...We had to be sure the door was closed while I was at the nursing home. Several times, she put a chair at the door so we wouldn't get surprised. Fortunately we didn't. We got our timing right. Lucky!*

*Doesn't that seem more positive? We're keeping depression at bay, hope alive and execution in play! There's the excuse. This is a way.*

*We are home. We don't have to worry about the nursing home door opening anymore.* Just reach out. With my disability, I had to be on the left side of the bed. We reached out to touch one another. Head, arms, legs, nothing sexual! Start the feelings. Kiss. Lightly run your nails gently over your partner's arms, their stomach, ever so slightly over their face and forehead and on to their scalp. Wherever. Don't have to go too far. At first, stay above the waist. Again, *One-step-at-a-time!* Leave it at that – a success.

Enjoy the feelings. The nursing home scene was better than nothing. This was clearly an improvement. More freedom! At home we could be more relaxed. It was wonderful to just feel something that felt good. And I was improving.

Not surprisingly, I was having lingering performance doubts. Women also! Can she get moist or lubricated? Turned on! Fair questions.

The caregiver, she's had her feelings bottled up during all of these months. Not terribly healthy. Begin her reawakening. At the beginning, start where it is comfortable! Touch, the right touch, very lightly. That can be electric!

Maybe a peck, better a French kiss and more stroking (no pun intended) and touching. Perhaps, not fully undressed at the beginning! For us, fully undressed, but every couple is different. You want the warmth; you want to stir some passion.

*No judgments here.*

Moving along at a non-threatening pace; or maybe faster, for others if it works for them. One step is more conservative. Touching first, later sexual touching but nothing more! Maybe repeat it. Another day, more active sexual touching! A future time, perhaps getting to climax with deeper kisses and so on!

What's the saying, learn to ride a bike once, you never forget!

**At a time like this we learned that the operable words are *thoughtful, mindful, sensitive and proactive*! Oh yes, get on with it! *We did.***

Most of us rode a bike in our youths or later. Let's go guys and gals - get a smile on!

*It takes two to tango!*

So at this juncture I thought readers would appreciate Debbie's comments on the two chapters on sex after stroke.

*Reflecting back, Debbie commented,*

*"Remember, we were only married eighteen months before Bob had his stroke. Like most newly married couples we had a healthy sex life, which with the stroke came to a screeching halt. We were in limbo on many things, and certainly sex was one of them. He was obviously in pretty bad shape so it would have been unreasonable for me to expect him to do much or take an initiation role in the sexual department. And certainly not in the nursing home!*

*But I yearned for the warmth, and I thought that some activity, whatever it was, would be good for him, and me. So I gradually took the initiative to start, as Bob described earlier!*

*I was glad I did, and though far from par, very far, his reactions made me feel better. And I quickly realized that it made him feel a bit more like himself. And as we progressed, I realized that over time we would be fine. To me, this was just one more thing that I, as the caregiver partner, had to get on top of!*

*And from my perspective, depending on the reader, I would think about doing the same, whatever it is. Something is better than nothing!"*

What can be...the delights? Using the One-step-at-a-Time Process! Think through a handicapped fix. What are the most doable and comfortable position(s) or which side of the bed works for the disabled partner. Admittedly, it's not as impromptu as it once was. But...

*Yes, there is beauty, life, intimacy and sex after stroke. Both of our lives have changed. True, it isn't the same as before, but then... embrace the New Us!*

# CHAPTER 38
# TRAVELING AFTER STROKE

---

*Debbie and I love to travel, and though I still am handicapped, we don't let that stop us.*

In December, 2012, we embarked on a six week journey all the way to Australia and New Zealand. Except for the cruise across the Tasmanian Sea to New Zealand we were on our own. And even then we planned independent excursions at each port except the last.

**PLANNING**

*Breaking down the barriers - my ankle*

Before we left, I started thinking about what would be the barriers to having a truly exceptional trip. Let's address them. The biggest issue was my weak right ankle which often prevents enjoyable walks, particularly on soft or uneven surfaces such as sand, grass, cobblestones and other rough surfaces. Situations I would undoubtedly I would have to deal with. This is frustrating, stressful, annoying and can be limiting.

But wait - I was watching the US Tennis Open and, lo and behold, I noticed that Andy Murray had an ankle brace that certainly seemed supportive, light weight and unobtrusive.

*"Doctor ......., Debbie and I are going to Australia in December for six weeks and I want to get Andy Murray's brace. We are going to be on tours and walking all over the place."*

He chuckled,

*"No I'm serious - I want Andy Murray's brace!"*

He referred me to a podiatrist in the hospital and I scheduled a visit.

Appraising me, "How can I help you?"

*"I want Andy Murray's brace for my right ankle"*

Likewise, she thought that I was kidding, but soon realized I was serious. So after examining my leg and ankle she Googled "Andy Murray's brace" and said,

*"Bob, I can't give you his brace but I can give you something that should do the trick."*

That weekend Debbie and I took to the beach for a dry run.

*I haven't walked on the beach like this for 17 years. Still not perfect, but a huge improvement.*

*Another barrier to consider- Wheelchairs in airports*

Traveling internationally often requires substantial walking in airports, security and customs clearances and a whole raft of other high energy and stressful activities. Though I don't like doing it, I often do use a wheelchair in airports on these longer trips at Debbie's insistence. In a smaller airport I rarely use them, but in airports like JFK or London's Heathrow we find its most prudent to utilize the services of a porter and wheel chair. The reality is that they squire you through the lines and customs clearances much more quickly, but that's not why I do it.

*I'd gladly stand in the lines and skip the handicaps. And we could always get the Global Entry Card which would also speed us through. Take the good with the bad.*

I find that it is best to get handicapped seating well in advance of the flight. Generally, this has required a call to the airline we are flying on, sometimes a few calls.

More recently with some of the airlines, I have noticed the distasteful tendency to charge for the more convenient seating for Debbie. For example, during our flights out to California to start our Australian journey, United gave me an Economy Plus seat which is where handicapped seating typically is, but they required us to pay an up-charge for Debbie to sit with me. I had some discussion with the airline about that but I ultimately paid for Debbie.

I have to say – *"United - bad form guys!"*

## AIRLINE AND HOTEL LOUNGES MAKE TRAVELING LESS STRESSFUL AND EASIER

Traveling, I also have found that the use of airline clubs like The Qantas Club make a world of difference, particularly on longer trips. When I am planning a trip, I will spend a bit of time strategizing how to get into these Clubs. Again, the devil's in the details and depending on the airline there can be arcane rules. Ways I have used to get free or discounted entry into airline clubs include specialty credit cards and airline alliance reciprocity agreements. For example, when flying Delta with a Delta branded American Express Card, I get 50 percent discounts at the Delta Sky Clubs.

Though I don't have one, I know that the American Express Platinum Card gets free entry into some of the Clubs. When going to Australia in the One World Alliance Family of Airlines we were able to use our American Airlines Admiral's Club membership to get free entry into the Qantas Clubs. Incidentally, be mindful that this could change with the US Air/American consolidation.

Similarly, with hotels, we more often than not try to stay in a hotel with a concierge lounge. It just makes it easier and I might add quite nice. We have free breakfast and often also have dinner in the lounge so that we don't have to go out again after a long day of touring. The room typically costs more but when you factor in the savings on food and wine the higher room cost is usually equalized, if not bettered. Most importantly I'm able to save some energy for the next day by using the Clubs. Admittedly we lose a bit of the local flavor by sometimes skipping the restaurants but you can't have everything!

## ELEVATOR ACCESS

Additionally, with lodging I will, without exception, look for a hotel with elevator access. But once in a while we can get surprised as we were in Amsterdam. In an older, well-cared for smaller hotel, there was an elevator. However, it didn't go all the way up to our room and, as luck would have it, there were no rooms with shower stalls available on the lower floors. So we toughed it for a few days and Debbie held on to me darn tightly. Frankly, it wasn't brilliant – there was a little more risk than we needed, but it worked out ok!

## ADA ROOMS

Depending on your situation, when considering a hotel you can require a handicapped accessible room, perhaps prefer one, but not require it, or, in my case, adamantly oppose it. Handicapped accessible rooms are typically in convenient locations near the elevator. As with everything, there is good and also bad! Convenience is good, however, in most hotels convenience comes with noise. Unless the hotel is built like Ft. Knox, the likelihood of hall noise trumps the convenience for us. ADA rooms are usually near the elevator with the potential for noisy revelers getting off the elevator. The first rooms they will pass are the ADA rooms. Then there is the issue of being next to the elevator shaft, with the potential for different noises and, finally, there are the conveniently located ice and snack machine rooms which can be right next door. Over the years we have experienced all of these situations, and more, so now we opt for a quiet room in a remote location and live with the longer walk.

## TRY FOR WALK-IN SHOWERS

I do, however, try to book a room with a walk-in shower. That can be easier said than done since many older hotels still have showers over tubs, even in the most upscale situations. At the newer, mid-priced hotels, they usually have showers over tub, think Hampton Inn, Hyatt Place, Marriott Courtyards and many others. However, if we are staying in a hotel where I think shower stalls are available, I may call the manager and explain my situation and ask for an accommodation.

If all else fails, I grab onto the fixtures or the bar that holds the shower curtain up to assist me as I enter and leave the shower. If Debbie is traveling with me, of course she steadies me if there isn't a place to hold on.

Another thing we do when traveling is to request a shower floor mat, particularly in a tub situation. We do the same in the case of the walk-in shower with a slippery tile floor. If it is not in our room a quick call to housekeeping usually solves the problem.

## TOURS

When we want to participate in a tour, I find that smaller group tours are more convenient for us. The smaller buses are often able to get closer to the destination and we are more often able to stay in the front few rows in a smaller, more intimate group. Also, the group is less likely to get away from us if it is smaller.

Finally, larger tours typically mean higher, more difficult-to-navigate bus entry stairs. The small group tours worked well for us in Australia. They also are more intimate.

## CRUISES

We have taken several cruises during the past few years. In general, they are handicap friendly. The crew can handle folks with wheel chairs and other disabilities. And there are elevators to assist in ship access. Finally, there are handicapped rooms with roll-in showers, etc. It just depends what is required to have a comfortable experience.

There are a few cautionary notes to consider as one selects the precise cruise to book. Based on my experience you might want to be mindful of any personal balance or vertigo issues and how they could be impacted by ship movement. I have described my balance problems and I can report that they can be an issue on a cruise, particularly on smaller ships in choppy waters. In general, larger, newer ships with stabilizers will have less movement. Also, I book staterooms nearer the middle of the ship. I have friends who book inside staterooms to alleviate the movement. This is all a personal decision, based on the needs and obviously the budget.

A second factor to investigate is the ports that the ship plans to visit. Will the ship be docked at the port so that there is a gang plank to utilize or will ship tendering be required? In the latter case, a handicapped person might want to skip that port, depending on the deficit. A friend of ours, now deceased, used to say, *"If I let all of this stop me, then I see zero, but if I skip one or two things and do everything else, I see 90% of what I wanted to see."* He and his wife went to China with that attitude and I totally agree.

Though we have never used one there are travel agents who specialize in disability travel. That could be helpful. I'd expect that professional to be knowledgeable about details of the various ships – how well stabilized, staterooms, locations, amenities, itineraries that are more handicapped friendly, etc.

**The take-away from all of this is: when traveling after Stroke or any other mobility disability, think it through, make a few extra calls and put in the extra time planning!**

# CHAPTER 39
# FITNESS AFTER STROKE

Udo Fischer, the psychologist I mentioned earlier said it, as have so many other healthcare professionals who agree - fitness and diet are key drivers to successful recovery. So when thinking about game changers after stroke these are critical factors; and I have certainly found this to be true. **I realized that if I was going to maximize my recovery it would be a lot easier if I was fit, at least as fit as I could be.** That's the case with both physical fitness, but also intellectual or brain fitness.

First physical, think about it! If I were to pick up a 25 pound cement block and carry it around, is it going to be easier or harder to do my tasks? If I have those 25 extra pounds on my body is it any different? My body has to work harder and it's more likely to break down. Why push it unnecessarily! It has already been rocked.

I am realistic and there are limits to what I can do to get myself physically fit; I'm still not going to run a marathon. One has to do what they can physically do in the context of their disabilities. And I might suggest proceeding one-step-at-a-time. There it is again!

I plan to work out just about every day; however, I find that business and social conflicts get in the way at least once per week. So six days a week is a serious commitment. Over the years, I've learned a few things about trying to be fit, not just thinking or talking about it, as many do.

By far the most important factor in my regular attendance at a fitness center is its convenience to either our home or work. When the fitness center is not convenient, I too often find excuses not to go. I don't think I am the only one.

Partner/spouse support and encouragement is also very constructive. I have to admit that knowing that Debbie, nine days out of ten, will inquire when I am exercising has been a positive factor in my regular exercise routine. When I am not exercising I get a funny look, so it's easier to just do it! Take my word! She walks the same walk. Only hers is longer, attending one to two hour-long exercise classes daily. She is really into it. I go for about 45 minutes to an hour.

With a disability I have found it is best to go to a fitness center affiliated with a hospital if one is available in your geography, as it is here in Naples. There are a few reasons. My observation is that hospital-affiliated centers tend to have more handicapped or user friendly equipment.

I always ride a recumbent bike for my aerobics. It's definitely best if those bikes have foot straps that are easily adjustable. Since my right foot is feeling challenged I like a foot strap so that my foot does not constantly slip off the pedal, thereby disturbing my exercise. In some facilities these straps are either not present or are hard to adjust, requiring attendant assistance. I've never had that problem in hospital-affiliated centers though admittedly my experience is narrow.

Another thing I particularly like in a facility is a padded stretching table, which also is more likely found in a hospital-affiliated center. That way I can do my important stretches without having to go down on the floor and then pull myself back up. Everyone needs to stretch, but even more so as we age or are disabled.

The fitness staff is another important consideration. I look for a CPR trained and certified staff member to be available at all times. Those folks should also be available to assist members without someone having to chase around the center looking for them.

For these reasons, I suggest a careful tour of any fitness center being considered, perhaps more than once. When I see prospective members on tour, I rarely see them being what I call, really observant. To be fair, those folks don't have my problems so they don't need to be as picky. The same could be said for me, prior to my having a stroke.

Now, I try the machines, not just look at them. Are they comfortable, easy to use, and clean? How many machines, if any, are out of order? Are there cleaning pads or liquids to use on the equipment? Is the locker room comfortable, sized properly to the membership and clean? Sized properly means the locker room is not a mad house at peak times, typically after 5 p.m. during the week and on Saturday mornings.

I've found that I go more often when there is some sense of camaraderie or friendliness in the facility, be it the staff or other members (my chattiness routine), or both.

*Something new*

I am not an exercise class person, preferring the machines. But recently I had occasion to learn of something called Chair Yoga. It was being demonstrated at the Brain Health Fair that I will discuss later. I watched Chair Yoga while I was talking to someone at the Fair, and *"I thought, I have to try this."* So I joined the demonstration group when my conversation ended.

Yoga moves are either performed sitting or behind or around a chair, which can be used for support and to assist with balance. I will be trying this form of yoga during the coming weeks, so admittedly this is a work in progress.

While I am on the subject of classes, I have started going to Balance classes to improve my balance. That's somewhat similar to the Yoga classes but there seems to be more of a specific balance focus. Again, a work in progress. Neither of these can hurt.

*I am always out there looking for something new. How about you?*

When we travel, we exercise, or at least we try. Some might find that a bit extreme but *it's a lifestyle thing for us.* So I look for hotels with fitness centers and, if Debbie is accompanying me, I also look for classes or a health club affiliation with classes so that she can do her thing while I use the machines. Likewise, if we are on a cruise we work out unless we have spent a really long day playing tourist.

We always feel better after exercising; it helps relieve stress, keeps us humming and burns calories, particularly when we travel.

A second dimension of fitness is brain fitness. Frankly, I have not considered this an issue being as mentally active as I have been over the past few years. In addition, the ETPS transformative moment that I described in Chapter 29 has made an enormous difference. But I have to admit that I could still improve and will spend some time in this area and perhaps blog about it.

Recently I attended a Brain Health Fair in Naples, FL, at NCH, a local hospital. Two speakers, an expert in health and rehabilitation psychology and a speech language pathologist discussed utilizing brain games to preserve and improve one's mental capacity. They were quite persuasive as brain games were described for use in improving problem solving, concentration and memory skills.

The speakers made reference to brain plasticity which is the same science that Dr. Edward Taub was concerned with when he developed Constraint Therapy (CI) and I have previously discussed.

Called a science of Neurobics, brain exercises and training are partnered with the consumption of brain foods. The speakers made mention of over 200 internet sites offering brain games but mentioned two in particular, Fit Brains and Lumosity. These two have interactivity and combine time limitations and rewards to encourage participation and long-term involvement. An audience member also mentioned PositScience as an alternative offering worth consideration.

For those less comfortable on the computer, there are alternative offline offerings. One that was suggested was The Brain Training Revolution by Paul Bendheim. That's more of a workbook.

*There is something profound here worth pursuing.*

# CHAPTER 40

# DIET AFTER STROKE

We also link exercise to diet as Udo said. The worsening obesity problem in our nation, and globally, has resulted in a higher incidence of diseases of the heart as well as diabetes. On the positive side there is starting to be more publicity to change one's eating habits.

The First Lady, Michelle Obama, has made it one of her important initiatives, particularly among school children. She is certainly on to something. If you can get kids to eat better they should have more healthy lives and hopefully have fewer strokes as they grow older. Then maybe they won't need this book -- a good thing!

For Debbie and myself, diet has always been important, even more so after my stroke. To the extent possible, we avoid salt, never adding it, all fast food, nearly all processed food, and foods with corn syrup. Due to this, I go to the supermarket four or five times a week to get fresh food, which admittedly is a nuisance. One thing that is nice though, is that many of the employees know me so the chattiness factor comes into play.

In an article in the Wall Street Journal on March 15, 2014, there was talk of an emerging partnership between some in the medical community and a group of chefs in the restaurant industry. That's really on target because much of the food served in restaurants contains unhealthy ingredients that I don't cook with such as salt, though I am aware that sea salt seems to be getting some positive buzz. The essence of the partnership is to serve healthy foods that taste appetizing so that more people eat in a healthy manner. They are trying to promote the idea that healthy foods are enjoyable to eat if properly prepared. Right on!

This group has developed something called Culinary RX which includes foods that are considered to be "recommended for eating well – in every sense." These include:

All kinds of green leafy vegetables
Onions
Whole grains
Seeds, dried beans and legumes
Mushrooms
Avocados
All kinds of berries
Stone fruit
Nuts and coconut
Eggs
Garlic
Olive oil
Wild salmon (not farm raised)
Organic chicken
Grass fed beef
Anchovies and sardines

*How many of these do you eat regularly? Or at all!*

We include as many of these suggested foods as possible in our diet, while also eating a wide variety of foods. The dinner salad recipe below is a perfect example. Though Debbie is not one to cook, (that's one reason she got interested in me since I do the cooking) she does make these huge dinner salads with all kinds of healthy ingredients. The salad which we have four or five days per week goes a long way to satisfy our hunger at dinner.

## DEBBIE'S GRAND DINNER SALAD

Mixed Greens – Various Lettuces, Arugula, Baby Spinach or Kale
Cut Celery
Cut Carrots
Tomato Chunks or Grape Tomatoes
Cucumber Slices

Fresh Avocado Pieces
Blueberries
Apple or Pear Chunks
Raspberries
Dried Cherries and Cranberries
Sliced Hard Boiled Eggs

We differ on a few other ingredients which I add including:

Strawberries
Fresh Pineapple
Melon Chunks
Green Pepper
Green Scallions

And she adds to hers

Large Green Olives
Artichokes in their oil which she uses as her salad dressing

Depending on how large a salad you prefer, and your tastes for each of these ingredients, the amounts of these ingredients will vary.

Chopped nuts, such as walnuts or almonds can also be added to this recipe. Preparation time for this salad is about 20-30 minutes depending on how fast you chop. If I did all of the chopping it would definitely take longer.

Sometimes Debbie will add grilled or rotisserie chicken, sliced flank steak or fresh shrimp. When she adds these latter ingredients, that's her dinner! I'm 95 percent vegetarian so I will often have some pasta in addition to the salad.

Since this salad is huge she serves it in a pasta bowl; otherwise the salad falls all over the place.

If she uses salad dressing, Debbie sticks to either Olive Oil or Balsamic Vinegar. I am not as disciplined. I like Marie's Cole Slaw

Dressing, Light Blue Cheese, Honey Mustard Dressing and Raspberry Vinaigrette. I also like Panera Bread Tangerine Vinaigrette and sometimes add crumbled fresh blue cheese.

I realize that some of my dressings violate what I previously said about processed foods; I'm not perfect. At other times, I dress my salad with light cottage cheese or balsamic dressing and crumbled blue cheese.

At festive times, I make my own salad dressing, a recipe from my cousin, Joyce:

> 1/4 cup Virgin Olive Oil
> 1 cup Balsamic Vinegar
> 3 or 4 Tablespoons Honey Mustard
> 1 Teaspoon – Dry Oregano
> ½ Teaspoon- Fresh Black Pepper
> ¼ Teaspoon Garlic Powder

Whisk all of these ingredients together ahead of time so that the flavors have a chance to meld. Re-whisk just before serving! Crumbled blue cheese is a nice complement to this dressing. Notice, I didn't add salt.

Preparation time for this salad dressing is five minutes and 30 seconds more before serving.

Bottom line for all of this focus on diet and exercise, my weight is at my post-basic training level, 48 years ago. Debbie is tiny.

## LOSING WEIGHT

Many people have asked how I have gotten my weight down and maintained it.

*A controversial approach that works for me*

One of the ways is to skip lunch or make it very small and nutritious.

That's what I do nine days out of ten. Skip. I recognize that this is difficult for many so it would have to be treated as a lifestyle change. Stay with me on this! To bridge the gap during the day, I will often have a few snacks such as a banana, other piece of fruit, perhaps some nuts, preferably the low sodium variety, a hand full or two of healthy trail mix or one or two mini-cookies. Never all of them!

Why skip? Lunches have tons of calories, which in my view should be avoided. It strikes me that virtually all fast food is either very high fat or very, very high fat. So, though not impossible, it's not easy to consistently find a healthy low-fat lunch.

I've also learned that by not eating too large a portion of food my stomach has gradually shrunk so I do not require that much to satisfy me at any meal. This is the natural way to reduce the size of one's stomach instead of risky surgery. But I'm not going to say this is easy at the beginning or for some, ever. And there are others who would say that it is unhealthy. I recognize that.

A trick I used, particularly at the beginning, was to substitute bottled lightly carbonated water like San Pellegrino or Perrier. The carbonation made me feel fuller. Sometimes I also have an iced coffee with non-fat milk and a sugar. I don't, but one could also drink a smoothie if it is made with healthy low-fat ingredients and limited sugar. That tends to be filling also.

I don't really understand why humans need three meals per day. People will say to me that they can't go more than a few hours without eating. But when you are sleeping you don't eat and if you wake up during the night, for whatever reason, it's a rare person who raids the refrigerator every night. Rather they go to the bathroom, read, and watch TV and hopefully then go back to sleep. So why not create a food gap during the day!

To accomplish the two-meal diet, I have a good breakfast and then a normal dinner. It's difficult to see how the two meal diet would work without a good breakfast. Breakfast consists of:

Oatmeal with dried cranberries,
Fresh cut apples, bananas and strawberries.
Half English muffin, bagel or small muffin
Hot or iced coffee

I sweeten the oatmeal with real maple syrup, not the fake stuff with corn syrup. A tip, get the real syrup in little jugs at Costco or Sam's Club, and it will cost less per ounce than the fake stuff in the supermarket. I looked at the labels of some of the syrups in the supermarket, and guess what? The ingredient list contained NO real syrup, only chemicals and corn syrup. Look at the ingredients in the fake stuff, then see if you want to eat that?

Some days instead of the oatmeal I have non-fat yogurt with granola or muesli, and the same fruit, to which I add blueberries. I sometimes have one or two pieces of fruit at lunch on those days since the yogurt is not as filling as the oatmeal. Other than that, I drink bottled water during the day. At dinner I have two glasses of wine. I'm allowed!

*Getting control of my weight has been important to my successful recovery. I have less to carry around. I'm not burning my energy on the wrong things.*

## SUPPLEMENTS

*Over the years, and today, I take a number of supplements to enhance my health. Everyone who takes supplements should do so with the input of their physician. You want to avoid drug interactions with any prescription medicine.*

Also, since supplements are not regulated in any substantial way, you want to purchase them from legitimate sources. Recently, there has been negative press about several of what I would have thought to be reliable sources who had supply issues. Care is advisable!

# Part VIII

# *Perspectives Moving Forward*

The future holds so much promise but only if we make it happen.

*-Bob Mandell*

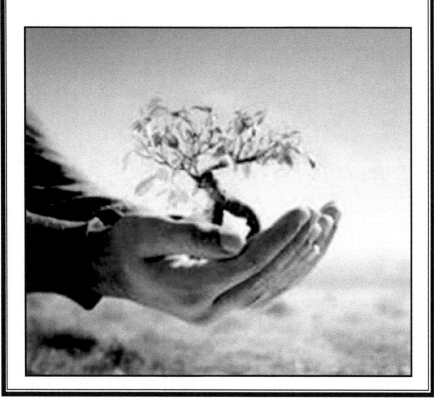

# CHAPTER 41

# TODAY'S HEALTHCARE – A SELF SERVICE MODEL

*It hit me like a ton of bricks – the new world of therapy, the whole new world of healthcare is a self-service model for most of us!*

I was reminded of an incident out of my past. In 1999, and recovering, I had been invited to a high level conference in Phoenix sponsored by the old US West Telecommunications Corporation. US West was the telecommunications provider in the Southwest portion of the US. One of the speakers, a futurist, was describing the new internet and how it would evolve.

He suddenly asked, *"What do you think the future internet business model is going to be?"* No one answered. He got several people on their feet and pressed for an answer in a probing manner, but no one had the right answer. Suddenly he was focused on me.

*Why me*
He put me on the spot by repeating his question. Not standing, as my public speaking persona was bad, I nervously answered as the whole room looked on,

*"That sounds like a self-service model,"* I managed to get out.

To which he enthusiastically said, "Right, now you've got it," as I took a deep breath of relief.

*"The internet is going to allow you and me to do so many things we couldn't do for ourselves"* he said excitedly. He was all for it.

2014 - Fast forward to healthcare today!

*I now think the same of the new healthcare environment, only; in this case it's not so good.* **To succeed in recovery from anything, we will have to be far more proactive, empowered and patient centric. We will have to take the bull by the horns.**

There are many terms, for example, US News and World Report in their Best Hospitals Issue termed it "Patient Power." Other writers call it "Patient Empowerment" or some such thing. Irrespective of what we label it, **we have entered an era where patients, and their caregivers, will have to take more responsibility for their healthcare decisions and therefore conduct more of their own due diligence. And with it, become self-advocates.** To be fair, the internet has given patients the tools to fulfill those roles. But still.

A recent experience confirmed my worst fears. Eight sessions of therapy for two broken vertebrae after surgery, was what was prescribed!

*Serious self-advocacy is required.*

Interestingly the need to conduct more self-directed treatment and therapy was recently confirmed while talking to a neurologist in Boca Raton where I was a participant in a clinical research study.

The neurologist commented, *"Patients don't realize it, but when therapy ends, that's just the beginning. They come in here, and they have completed their therapy and are not continuing to exercise or stretch or do anything else to keep going. And they are frustrated and have symptomatic complaints. You have done something else. You keep your treatments going without being told and look at you now."*

The New Healthcare- self-educated, directed, and advocated.

**A self-service model!**

# CHAPTER 42

# STROKE VICTORS HAVE A STROKE READINESS PLAN: *DO YOU?*

*"All hospitals are not created the same."* Dr. *Nasser Razack, Lee Memorial Health System*

Living in Florida, Debbie and I have a hurricane readiness plan. It's prudent! As July rolls around we stock up on drinking water and batteries for flashlights. We have a radio powered by batteries to get emergency news. We are aware of the automobile escape route. Some get or check their power generators. A plan, whatever it is!

*But isn't stroke more serious? This is a disease where minutes wasted means brain loss!*

So with stroke, how many also have a readiness plan? I would bet, damn few! Out of curiosity, I asked a friend who goes regularly to my fitness center if he had a stroke plan. He looked at me quizzically. Mind you, this is a very successful, educated and experienced former executive, now retired. No dope! Likewise, I will readily admit to not having a plan in 1996 when I had my stroke. "It can't or wouldn't happen to me!" Well, we know that's BS!

But, thinking about it – a disease of seconds and minutes which stroke is; a disease where "time loss is brain loss". A plan to save time is critical. And the plan can't be to Google "stroke hospital" while EMS is sitting in the driveway!

*So do you have a stroke plan?*

I recently attended a presentation by Dr. Nasser Razack, a neurointerventional radiologist at Lee Memorial Health System in Ft. Myers, Fl. The major take-away from the presentation:

## HAVE A STROKE READINESS PLAN!

*What does it entail? And besides time saved, why might I need it?*

The simple answer is embodied in the quote above – *"all hospitals are not created the same"*. Every hospital has its own strengths and weaknesses. The level of care that they are capable of successfully delivering by disease varies. Some may be strong in diseases of the heart, or diabetes, or obstetrics. Whatever! Or they are small community hospitals where they can't afford the medical infrastructure to properly treat something as complex as stroke. Or they are big multi-location hospitals with only one Stroke Center. There are many scenarios.

**The most important part of the stroke plan is to know how to advocate for the best care, <u>in detail</u>.** Dr. Razack made the point that in the case of a stroke, you really want to be taken initially and immediately to a hospital capable of administering a rapid assessment and initial clot busting drugs. That initial treatment is very important because 1.9 MILLION brain cells die each MINUTE during a stroke.

After the initial treatment, it is then very important to advocate for yourself, or if you are the caregiver partner, the patient. The critical step is to request an evaluation for additional treatment at a Stroke Center **"with all the bells and whistles"**. (Note: if the patient is one of the 15% of patients who suffer a brain bleed, known as a Hemorrhagic Stroke, as I had, the Stroke Center will first stabilize them and then perform neurosurgery to repair the bleed.)

Let me briefly describe the Stroke Center landscape so that you have an initial understanding of the differences. There are two types of certifications that a Stroke Center can have from two entirely different kinds of certifiers. First, each State, typically the States' Department of Health, certifies hospital stroke centers based on the medical skill sets embodied in the hospital's Stroke Team. That's pretty straight forward.

In Florida, as in other states, there are two levels of Centers – Comprehensive and Primary, though the names might be different in various States. The difference between the two types of centers is the amount and type of interventions that the hospital can provide. The Comprehensive Center, of which there are only about thirty in Florida, can provide the fullest range of interventions. These are the Centers with "all the bells and whistles" to use Dr. Razack's words. But they aren't available in all geographies or they may not be the closest Stroke Center to the patient.

The Primary Center, of which there are more, can provide some, but not all interventions. In larger hospital systems one location may be certified as a Comprehensive Center, while other locations are certified as Primary Centers, and then other locations may have no certification at all. Beyond a shadow of doubt, some is very much better than none.

The second type of certifiers are voluntary organizations such as the Joint Commission on Accreditation of Healthcare Organizations (JCAHO) and DNV Healthcare which focus on quality driven accreditation and clinical excellence hospital certifications, safety, cleanliness and staff knowledge ability skill sets, among others.

For example, the Joint Commission website states,

*"The Joint Commission accredits and certifies more than 20,500 health care organizations and programs in the United States. Joint Commission accreditation and certification is recognized nationwide as a symbol of quality that reflects an organization's commitment to meeting certain performance standards."*

This dual certification - State and voluntary certifiers is interesting, but a little much certainly to the non-medically trained person. This is particularly the case when hospitals advertise their certifications, as they do in my geography.

Let's look at a few examples and I will use my geography to illustrate. Lee Memorial Health System has four adult acute care hospitals in and surrounding the city of Ft. Myers and Lee County, where Ft. Myers is located. However, only the Gulf Coast Medical Center is a Comprehensive Stroke Center. A few of the other locations are Primary Centers and one is "Stroke Ready", a lesser designation. Lee Memorial has a "hub and spoke" concept. The Comprehensive Stroke Center serves as a "hub" for the Primary Stroke Centers to send patients for advanced treatment.

In Florida, and in many, but not all States, EMS operates using protocols that direct transport of stroke patients to designated stroke centers whenever possible. The important thing to do is to dial 911 and allow EMS to transport the patient to the closest appropriate facility. Remember "time is brain!" After the initial assessment and treatment you, acting for yourself or your caregiver partner will want to insist that the patient is evaluated for additional treatment at an appropriate hospital, a facility that you know has the most comprehensive stroke capabilities in the geography.

To further illustrate, let's look at a few common stroke situations. The three-hour clot busting medication intervention can be provided at the Comprehensive Stroke Centers and the Primary Stroke Centers, or at general hospitals. However, many serious larger vessel situations which often result in death or long-term disability require more aggressive interventions that are only available at a Comprehensive Stroke Center. In those latter cases, the patient at a Primary Stroke Center must be transferred to the more comprehensive facility by helicopter or ambulance depending on the geography in question. These patients may still have clot(s) remaining in the vessel that the clot busting medicine could not dissolve.

Just out of curiosity, I tried my earlier question on another friend. Having breakfast with a very intelligent practicing attorney, actually a Partner in a very fine firm, I asked him the same question - where would you go? Initially, his first response was *"I have no clue."* As we talked a bit more he said, *"I guess Health Park."* To which I said, *"Wrong…"* It shook him! Actually, Health Park is "stroke ready" which is a lower designation.

We are not through! So, let's say you have taken my suggestion and are earnestly trying to find a Stroke Center in your geography.

To start the search for the correct Center in your geography you might go to the Internet Stroke Center at www.strokecenter.org. On their home page they have a link to their stroke center database, among other things. Their database seems quite comprehensive however please do not solely rely on it. That is because it utilizes the JCAHO data base but as I pointed out earlier, JCAHO is not the only certifying agency. For example, Lee Memorial Health System in Lee County, FL is certified by DNV Healthcare (www.dnvglhealthcare.com). And other Centers may not be certified by either because, remember, it is voluntary.

The JCAHO certified center which came up in my zip code search was NCH-Downtown, who were Primary Certified but who has just recently achieved the Florida State Comprehensive Stroke License.

Which brings up another point – sometimes there are changes in designations as in NCH which recently achieved the higher Comprehensive Stroke Center designation. It can go the other way also. It appears that Physicians Regional, in Naples FL, will be losing their Comprehensive Stroke Center in April 2015.

I decided to perform the same search, only this time, in Connecticut where Debbie and I lived before moving to Florida. Going back to the Internet Stroke Center website – www.StrokeCenter.org because it's easier to navigate, I put in a zip code in downtown Stamford – 06901.

The only Comprehensive Stroke Center I could find was in Hartford which I found remarkable. Hartford Hospital, where the Center is located is over one hour driving time from Stamford, without traffic which isn't very often. Anybody who drives Connecticut knows what I am referring to. Perhaps they do helicopter transports. Hartford Hospital was quite proud of their dual certification based on the press release they put out in 2013 when they achieved the certifications.

Then I went to the Connecticut Department of Public Health website. I found a list of 22 Primary Stroke Centers which span the State. Cross checking the JCAHO list, I found that only nine of them are JCAHO certified. In my search using Stamford, the data base identified several Primary Stroke Centers, two of which were within ten miles of 06901. I also checked if any of the Stroke Centers in Connecticut were DNV certified but none were.

The situation in the nation as a whole is no less confusing. With respect to other States, one might want to investigate the definitions, designations and locations of Stroke Centers in your geography. This way you will not mix up the designations and possibly confuse the EMS personnel.

**This is just another case in the medical field where self-advocacy and education is prudent. What all of this suggests is the need for prior research on the nearest location of a Comprehensive Center, and also as a Plan B, the nearest Primary Stroke Center.**

In the pressure of the moment coming up with a stroke center, or the right stroke center is highly problematic. The implications could be very significant, life threatening at the extreme, and certainly lifestyle threatening due to the disabilities, post-stroke.

*It's time to consult your physician, make it part of your plan! Before the fact!!*

Now you might have thought to yourself, why is Bob putting me through all of this confusion? I'll just ask my doctor. And that's fine as long as you do it before the event! But there is a concept in medicine called the Informed Patient. I have always had much more constructive conversations with healthcare professionals when I did my homework first.

*If this long chapter has made you think to ask your Doctor for a recommendation before the fact or make the determination independently, then I am satisfied that I have achieved my objective.*

In speaking with your physician, ask where would they go with their family, given your geography? See if you can make a determination, and then get it confirmed. And what if you are traveling? Now at least you know the right questions. Enough!

To get back to the readiness plan, as I said earlier **use the services of 911** rather than driving or having someone drive the patient to the Emergency Room. EMS has knowledge, can move faster and start the evaluation while in transit. There is some new telemedicine technology that is being integrated into protocols which can speed diagnosis and which could make a difference to long term stroke outcomes.

Your plan might also include some research regarding the backgrounds of the physicians – neurosurgeons, neurologists and cardiologists at the Stroke Center as well as post-surgery physicians. If this is your first go-round with stroke, what do you know about physicians in these specialties? We didn't!

Another item your Stroke Readiness Plan might include is a **Completed Medical Register** for each person in your residence. I was given one at a stroke presentation at Physicians Regional. Their register folds to 2x3, business card size and fits in a little plastic case.

Included on the information to be filled out <u>upon receipt</u> so it's ready, just in case:   Name,
                  Address,
                  Phone number, mobile, home, office
                  Date of birth,
                  Blood type,
                  Social security number,
                  Allergies and conditions,
                  Prescription medications with strength and dosage,
                  Emergency names and phone numbers,
                  Doctor's names and phone numbers,
                  Insurance information.

<u>**Finally, before I end this chapter, may I strongly suggest everyone reading this book carefully review and understand the information in Appendix III regarding Stroke Signs and**</u>

**<u>Symptoms and the F.A.S.T. quick risk factor system, provided by the CDC - NIH website.  That is also part of the readiness plan.</u>**

*Stroke Victors and their caregivers are informed patients! They have a Stroke Readiness Plan!*

*Other diseases!*

Note: Stroke is not the only disease that requires a Plan. Diligence should be implemented for other diseases, particularly if there is family history and they are catastrophic. This is especially important if the disease, like stroke, comes upon you suddenly like a heart attack.

From a hospital perspective, a broad resource is the *US News and World Report*, Top Hospitals Edition, which is updated annually.

Finally, if your local hospital has an active Outreach Program, may I suggest that you take advantage of it and become familiar with their services and facilities.

# CHAPTER 43

# A BREATH OF FRESH AIR – NIH STROKENET

Writing this book, I have come to realize that the amount of stroke research, particularly privately funded research, currently conducted is underwhelming, given the number of people who are impacted one way or another by the disease. That needs to change.

As a patient in several research studies I have also concluded that there is a need to speed up the research process without any deleterious impacts on the science being studied.

It is with profound delight that I recently read in *NeurologyNow* (April/May 2014) that the National Institute of Neurological Disorders and Stroke (NINDS), a part of the National Institutes of Health (NIH) has created something called NIH StrokeNet.

*"NINDS believes that NIH StrokeNet can accelerate the search for better ways to prevent, treat and recover from strokes while at the same time reducing redundant costs."* According to Dr. Walter J. Koroshetz, NINDS Deputy Director and a Fellow of the American Academy of Neurology, "NIH StrokeNet will allow the most promising therapies to quickly advance to the clinic – to improve prevention, acute treatment, or rehabilitation of the stroke patient."

A network of 25 Regional Coordinating Stroke Centers, plus satellite hospitals strategically located across the nation will coordinate stroke trials and research. In addition, an effort will be made to streamline the administration of the studies to reduce redundant efforts in the areas of trial infrastructure, trial agreements, contracts and protocols.

From my experiences, I can imagine many ways to speed the process and have developed what I call *A Patient Perspective*.

Furthermore, with the publication of this book, I, in cooperation with other concerned citizens are creating a Foundation to raise funds in the private sector to increase Stroke Research as will be more fully described later in this book.

*It's all very exciting and about time!*

Efforts will also be made to get patients more easily involved in the process. According to Dr. Petra Kaufmann, Director of NINDS Office of Clinical Research, *"Trials are the best way to evaluate new therapies. However, in order to conduct them in a timely manner we need more people to volunteer."* I've been saying that. Let's do our part to make it happen!

I wrote about that in my earlier chapters, trying to demystify the Clinical Research process and discussing the opportunities for patients. Participating in this process is the Dessert in my Chinese Family Dinner described in Chapter 22.

But don't wait to get going as NIH StrokeNet will take some time to be fully functional and I am sure there are opportunities this very day.

To keep informed of progress please visit www.StrokeVictor.com and opt-in to our email list.

# CHAPTER 44

# LAST BUT NOT LEAST, MY SECRET INGREDIENTS!

It's April, 2014, at the end of one of our sessions for my shoulder. I am slowly getting up from the stretching table at Physician's Regional Physical Therapy Center. My back was bothering me. I winced. Katie inquired, "You all right?"

*"My back is bothering me from lying on the table. I still can't get my back brace on to give it the support it needs." "Are you doing your back exercises?"* she inquired. *"What I can, with my shoulder restrictions, you know me."*

Gazing at her, "You know Katie, *I'm just a mule, and I just keep going, pain or no pain!"*

With a twinkle in her eye, Katie shot back, *"You know Bob, that's your real secret. You just keep at it! Put that on the last page of your book. End with your secret ingredients!"*

"Great idea, Katie!" The recipe is:

## One part each of, Grit, Moxie, Tenacity, and Endurance
## Topped off with a splash of
## Stubborn Mule

**Blend them all together and you get,**

## "STROKE VICTOR"

# AND THAT CAN BE <u>YOU</u> TOO!

## YOU AND YOURS CAN BE STROKE VICTORS!

### <u>JOIN THE STROKE VICTOR COMMUNITY</u>

*"The only courage you ever need is the courage to live the life you want."*

*—Oprah Winfrey*

# *Afterword*

## *Advocacy*

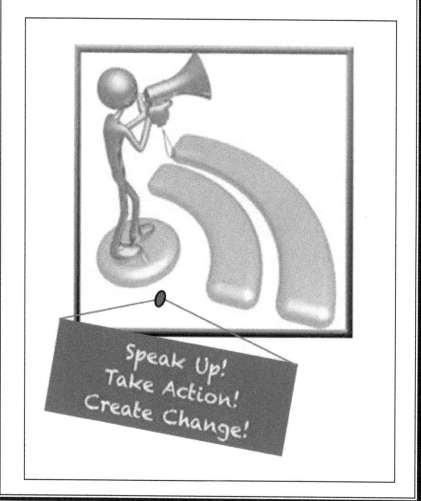

Speak Up!
Take Action!
Create Change!

# AFTERWORD - ADVOCACY

# THE STROKE RESEARCH FOUNDATION

*Recovering from my stroke, I had no idea of the seriousness of the problem- Stroke is underserved. Big time - It's time to fix it!*
*--Bob Mandell*

One of my primary objectives in writing this book was to provide a platform to speak about, and advocate for more focus on stroke. Much more! Meeting with scientists and medical professionals who have something to do with stroke, I frankly, became appalled and more than a little, astounded.

## Stroke is an amazingly underserved disease!

Below, I describe the broad elements and reasons for The Foundation I have established to focus on this monumental disease.

**The Stroke Research Foundation**, a charitable 501c3 organization dedicated to raising money to fund Stroke Research with the objective of improving stroke rehabilitation and recovery outcomes – faster and more complete. It's about substantially improving lifestyles, sooner rather than later!

This will profoundly help many people, not only the survivors but their caregivers and those in their extended communities. Take it from me, when stroke hits a family, there is considerable "people collateral damage".

*Here are some uncomfortable facts for background!*

Currently there are nearly 800,000 strokes occurring annually in the US with millions more people, who, like me, are living with the after-effects of earlier strokes.

As the projected baby-boomer demographics become a reality, our nation will be populated with a larger number of individuals 65 and older. It is not unreasonable to expect those numbers to climb to over one million new diagnoses annually. Likewise, the survivor figures will grow to eight to ten million. And these numbers are only for the United States.

Another disturbing fact and one that is a primary reason for The Foundation's existence:

**Today, stroke is the number one long-term disabler!!**

**As a stroke survivor, and author of this book, I believe the field of stroke is dramatically underserved in awareness, education, research dollars, singularly focused healthcare personnel, and privately funded development and fund raising efforts.**

There is a perception by many that Stroke is an elder disease. While partly true, that notion does not tell the entire story, far from it. **34%\* of new diagnoses are in people under 65, as I was.** And today, as many of us know, 65 is the new 50! **Many survivors are in their forties and fifties or younger.** Surprising to many, children can also have strokes. I recently met a lovely woman whose baby had a stroke and ultimately passed away.

The disease is highly complex in that there are many types of strokes. Furthermore, no two strokes are alike and no two outcomes are the same, all of which has serious implications for stroke rehabilitation and recovery. It is a "bespoke" disease—interesting in that something "bespoke," is differentiated, unique and custom which is typically associated with excellence--a custom-built car, a custom-fitted English suit. With stroke, it's quite the opposite—"custom" means it's difficult, time consuming and often expensive to treat.

While there are many cardiologists and neurologists, many of whom treat other significant diseases of the brain and heart, there's no such thing as a "strokeologist." Actually, that's my word!

What is missing then is a substantial body of healthcare clinicians and researchers, **<u>appropriate to the size of the problem</u>** and the number of new diagnoses, who are unwavering in their commitment to understand, treat and cure the disease called stroke. This will take time, serious advocacy and funding of research. **And it will take a shift in perception—from stroke victim to stroke victor!**

**For anyone who addresses and beats stroke, and anyone involved in helping others to beat stroke truly is a "Stroke Victor."** Let's join together and conquer stroke once and for all.

The Stroke Research Foundation will play a leading and critical role in addressing this gaping need. Just how you may ask!

First, we will fund patient centric innovative research focused on improved rehabilitation – new options and practical 21$^{st}$ Century approaches that can be implemented in the near-term;

Second with respect to improved post-stroke lifestyles, we will communicate in non-technical terms the results of research we fund, as well as others, so that survivors, caregivers and their tribes can visualize the opportunities. If the survivor or caregiver partner does not know of the innovation, what good is it?

And over time we will develop additional innovative initiatives such as a stroke mentorship program to encourage young researchers to commit to stroke research.

All focused on improving stroke lifestyles - NOW

*The Foundation needs YOUR help to serve the broad Stroke Community!*

*I hate to say it, but the lifestyle improvements your dollars help to fund, may be your own!*

*Donations are thankfully accepted on The Foundation website www.StrokeRF.org.*

---Bob Mandell

* Johns Hopkins Medicine

# *Resources*

**Infinite resources are global.**
- *Bob Mandell*

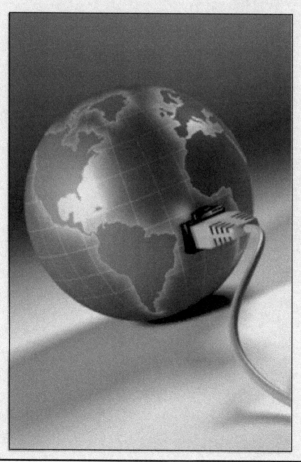

# APPENDIX AND RESOURCES

I - DEBBIE'S CRITERIA FOR A LIVE – IN REHABILITATION CENTER

II - WHAT MAKES A GREAT RECOVERY TEAM

III - WHAT YOU MAY NOT WANT TO KNOW BUT <u>NEED</u> TO KNOW - SOME STROKE FACTS OF LIFE

IV – THE GAME-CHANGERS

# APPENDIX I

# DEBBIE'S CRITERIA FOR A LIVE-IN REHABILITATION CENTER

1 - <u>Acceptance of our insurance.</u>

This is a pretty obvious issue for nearly everyone except perhaps the so-called 1% who might be willing to spend their own money to get what they want. The numbers can get substantial in the case of stroke. In today's insurance environment most policies have limits to the number of days in residence and the amount of rehabilitation therapy that will be approved for payment.

2 - <u>Convenience of facility to where Debbie worked so she could visit daily.</u>

Debbie had a busy work schedule but still wanted to visit daily. She also correctly believed that I would not do well if I felt isolated. I think the same can be said for anyone so long as they are in some kind of reasonable relationship.

3 - <u>Convenience to friends and family so that I would have regular visitors.</u>

Similarly, it would be important for her family and our friends to visit often, at least partly to jog my speech and to alleviate boredom to the extent possible.

4 - <u>Cleanliness of facility and equipment.</u>

Clearly one would want a clean facility that does not smell as some nursing homes do. The facility does not need to be new but being more modern can sometimes help. Not to be overlooked is regular cleaning of the rehab equipment which is getting used daily and therefore being touched by different people constantly. Cleanliness rules!

5 - Qualifications and attitude of PT, OT and Speech therapy staff or staff for whatever therapy might be required.

We were both determined that I get better. To accomplish that task one needs caring and excellent therapy from the professional staff. Certainly an excellent way to assess that is the qualifications of the staff.

Staff attitude is equally important and that's best determined by visits, and if you can get them, patient (or their caregiver or partner) references on the staff. Also if possible, observing the staff working with other patients and chatting with them to make your own assessment.

Debbie focused on how the staff was working with the patients or if they were otherwise preoccupied with paperwork or talking among themselves. They could be talking to one another or doing paperwork while the patient is doing an unsupervised activity which means that they might be doing it incorrectly, or the "easy way."

6 - Resident Profile – Men in attendance, age of residents.

Debbie wanted to be sure that there were other male patients, given the demographics of older patients.

7 - Was therapy implemented in groups or on a one-to-one basis?

Debbie visited several facilities that held group therapy sessions. To succeed, she believed that most if not all therapy should be individualized in order to get the best outcomes, certainly in my case. Every patient is different and individualized therapy accommodates that fact. While others might do well in a group setting, and that works for them, it would not work for me.

8 - <u>Private Room available with phone.</u>

Eighteen years ago was a different time in the insurance reimbursement world, so, a private room was doable with excellent insurance. Sadly, it is not necessarily doable today with most insurance contracts! However, if this is important, see if the facility will allow you to just pay the up-charge from a semi-private room to a private accommodation.

9 - <u>Friendliness, caring attitude and flexibility of the administrative staff.</u>

Though the administrative staff plays a behind the scene role, Debbie correctly believed that an excellent relationship can often result in a better experience for both patient and patient advocate/caregiver.

Perhaps, I should comment about the criteria. Debbie used the criteria that she developed as a way of thinking and viewing each of the seven facilities during that long day in February 1996. But every patient and situation is different. So, while the categories that she used would be important to anyone in the caregiver position, the answers could certainly be different for each family situation.

As one thinks about these criteria one could easily have selected a different facility and been right for their situation. For example, some patients might do well in a group therapy set-up, preferring the group camaraderie. Others, might not mind having a shared room or not have the insurance coverage for a private room.

There are as many scenarios as there are patients.

# APPENDIX II

# WHAT MAKES A GREAT RECOVERY TEAM

I've learned that stroke comes in many flavors and intensities. Dr. Eskioglu Director, Stroke and Neurovascular Surgery at Physician's Regional Hospital in Naples commented to me that "no two strokes are the same nor are no two outcomes." From the minor to the massive and everything in between! And with that, survivors have many variations in the types and seriousness of the resulting deficits to be addressed. Hence, my recovery team may not be another person's recovery team.

That said, beating the odds after stroke requires some or all of the following professionals to be part of the team.

## Physicians

Internist - specializes in overall patient health and in today's healthcare insurance environment, is often the gatekeeper for more advanced services. We have had considerable positive experience with these physicians.

Cardiologist - specializes in diseases of the heart. After my stroke, I had high blood pressure that needed stabilizing. I learned that the process of regulating the heart is both scientific and an art. It took months and many trials and errors to put together the right combination of pharmaceuticals to finally get my blood pressure under control.

Ultimately it was a nephrologist, who also worked in the cardiology field, to come up with the Catapres Patch solution, which in combination with some oral pharmaceuticals provided a successful long-term solution.

Neurologist - specializes in brain disorders including stroke. Though I saw several neurologists, I don't remember them making much of an impact. That's me, I am sure other survivors have had other experiences.

Neurovascular Surgeon – provides the surgical interventions should they be required after a patient suffers a stroke. This is critical, particularly during the early stage.

Physiatrist - specializes in rehabilitation. I saw several who made many positive suggestions as to facilities to go to for rehabilitation services. They also suggested practical things such as numbers of visits and for what services, in addition to writing the scripts for those services. I have been plagued with neck pain and it was a physiatrist who gave me cortisone shots to alleviate the pain. Unfortunately, though I had short term relief, it only lasted for a few months after each shot. I stopped having the shots.

Neuropsychologist – specializes in brain-related psychological conditions such as memory, behavior and thinking changes. I never was treated by one of these specialists though, for others, they could be very important.

Psychologist - specializes in emotional and behavioral conditions stemming from brain disorders. Soon after my stroke and during my early outpatient therapy days, I was treated a few times by a psychologist.

Optometrist - specializes in eye care. I had a significant vision and perceptual loss on my right side, which needed correction before I could return to driving. Until I had the driver evaluation, I was not aware of the loss.

## **Therapists and other healthcare professionals**

Physical Therapists (PT) - specialize in body movements like balance, walking, gait, stair walking and standing. They also focus on muscle strengthening and the use of aids such as canes. I had, and still have physical therapy, to improve my strength and walking ability. My experiences, with just a few brief exceptions were positive, some remarkable.

Occupational Therapists (OT) - specialize in activities of daily living such as body hygiene, dressing, eating, cooking and writing. They also focus on post - stroke living. I have had considerable positive experience with OT's.

Speech Therapists or Speech Pathologists - specialize in communication skills such as speaking and reading. They also assist with swallowing issues. I worked with several speech therapists that assisted with my speaking skills which I needed to relearn early in my recovery.

Social Worker - provides assistance with issues such as future living arrangements including such areas as rehab programs, living arrangements, at home living support and insurance aspects. Debbie had a small amount of positive experience with social workers. In other family situations, they may play a larger role.

Case Manager - specializes in coordinating care and providers. We had no experience with case managers since Debbie in the early years, and I later, performed this function. A case manager may have played a behind the scenes role at the nursing home where I was at the beginning of my recovery.

Dietician - specializes in advising on diet and healthy eating. That means for example, low salt and fat foods. In the nursing home we had a bit of experience with a dietician because I wanted my lunches to be fruit salads. They also advised on my other meals. Going forward, they are a very constructive part of a recovery team since healthy eating is critical to recovery.

Fitness Professional – specializes in advising on an appropriate fitness regimen and then possibly supervising the implementation of the program. During my out-patient therapy years in Connecticut I worked extensively with an exercise physiologist team who designed a fitness program for me and then supervised it.

Upon joining fitness center there are typically one or several introductory sessions with a personal trainer to familiarize the member with the facilities and the various machines. In addition, the trainer should create a chart with personalized settings on each machine for each member.

A disabled person will want to work with someone who is sensitive to their deficits and creates a fitness plan that will maximize their potential gains while not overdoing it.

## Stroke Coach

Assist the caregiver and survivor with issues of personal advocacy to get the correct resources, identification of recovery and rehabilitation resources, creation and guidance in the execution of a multidisciplinary stroke recovery plan to include all required aspects, navigating the clinical research system if the patient were interested, and last but not least, a friendly ear to add input and perspective, from someone who has "walked the walk".

Can we be helpful?

Reach us at bob@strokevictor.com

# APPENDIX III

# WHAT YOU MAY NOT WANT TO KNOW BUT *NEED TO KNOW*

## SOME STROKE FACTS OF LIFE

This book focuses on "after stroke." However, I believe that many readers will be, or are caregivers, family and other interested parties who have not themselves had a stroke.   The overall stroke community is huge.

*I want to keep it that way and take my word – so do you!*

For that reason, I have assembled some critical facts FROM THE U.S. Government Centers for Disease Control (CDC) website including stroke risk factors and symptoms to read, digest and be alerted to. This includes adapting a healthy lifestyle.

*My lifestyle chapters were not just for the stroke survivor.*

Here's some ugly statistics:
- Stroke kills almost **130,000** Americans each year—that's **1 out of every 19 deaths.**[1]
- On average, one American dies from stroke every **4 minutes.**[2]
- Every year, more than **795,000 people** in the United States have a stroke.
- About 610,000 of these are first or new strokes.
- About 185,00 strokes—**nearly one of four**—are in people who have had a previous stroke.[2]
- About **87%** of all strokes are ischemic strokes, when blood flow to the brain is blocked, a clot.[2]
- Stroke costs the United States an estimated **$36.5 billion** each year.[2] This total includes the cost of health care services,

medications to treat stroke, and missed days of work.
- Stroke is a leading cause of serious long-term disability.[2]

Stroke Risk Varies by Race and Ethnicity

Stroke is the fifth leading cause of death for Americans, but the risk of having a stroke varies with race and ethnicity. Risk of having a first stroke is **nearly twice** as high for blacks than for whites, and blacks are **more likely to die** following a stroke than are whites.[2] Hispanics' risk for stroke falls between that of whites and blacks.[2] American Indians, Alaska Natives, and blacks are more likely to have had a stroke than are other groups.[3]

# Stroke Signs and Symptoms

Sudden severe headache with no known cause is an important stroke sign in men and women.

*Remember, that's what I had.*

During a stroke, every minute counts! Fast treatment can reduce the brain damage that stroke can cause.

By knowing the signs and symptoms of stroke, you can be prepared to take quick action and perhaps save a life—maybe even your own. Watch a video about stroke signs and symptoms from the National Institute of Neurological Disorders and Stroke. (www.ninds.nih.gov/)

Signs of Stroke in Men and Women

- Sudden **numbness** or weakness in the face, arm, or leg, especially on one side of the body.
- Sudden **confusion**, trouble speaking, or difficulty understanding speech.
- Sudden **trouble seeing** in one or both eyes.
- Sudden **trouble walking**, dizziness, loss of balance, or lack of coordination.
- Sudden **severe headache** with no known cause.

References

1. Kochanek KD, Xu JQ, Murphy SL, Miniño AM, Kung HC. Deaths: final data for 2009. [PDF-371K] *Nat Vital Stat Rep.* 2011; 60(3).
2. Go AS, Mozaffarian D, Roger VL, Benjamin EJ, Berry JD, Borden WB, et al. Heart disease and stroke statistics—2013 update: a report from the American Heart Association. *Circulation.* 2012:e2–241.

## Acting F.A.S.T. Is Key for Stroke

Acting F.A.S.T. can help stroke patients get the treatments they desperately need. The most effective stroke treatments are only available if the stroke is recognized and diagnosed within three hours of the first symptoms. Stroke patients may not be eligible for the most effective treatments if they don't arrive at the hospital in time.

If you think someone may be having a stroke, act F.A.S.T.[1] and do the following simple test:

**F—Face:** Ask the person to smile. Does one side of the face droop?
**A—Arms:** Ask the person to raise both arms. Does one arm drift downward?
**S—Speech:** Ask the person to repeat a simple phrase. Is their speech slurred or strange?
**T—Time:** If you observe any of these signs, call 911 immediately.

**Note the time when any symptoms first appear.** Some treatments for stroke only work if given in the first three hours after symptoms appear. Do not drive to the hospital or let someone else drive you. Call an ambulance – 911 so that medical personnel can begin life-saving treatment on the way to the emergency room.

Treating a Transient Ischemic Attack

If your symptoms go away after a few minutes, you may have had a transient ischemic attack (TIA). Although brief, a TIA is a sign of a serious condition that will not go away without medical help. Tell your healthcare team about your symptoms right away.

Unfortunately, because TIAs clear up, many people ignore them. Don't be one of those people. Paying attention to a TIA can save your life.

The above data was taken from the CDC website and is public domain information.

## References

1.  National Institute of Neurological Disorders and Stroke. Brain Basics: Preventing Stroke Accessed December 4, 2013.

### Preventing Stroke: Healthy Living

Physical activity can help you maintain a healthy weight and lower cholesterol and blood pressure.

You can help prevent stroke by making healthy lifestyle choices. A healthy lifestyle includes the following:
- Eating a healthy diet.
- Maintaining a healthy weight.
- Getting enough exercise.
- Not smoking.
- Limiting alcohol use.

## Healthy Diet

Choosing healthy meal and snack options can help you avoid stroke and its complications. Be sure to eat plenty of fresh fruits and vegetables.

Eating foods low in saturated fats, Trans fat, and cholesterol and high in fiber can help prevent high cholesterol. Limiting salt (sodium) in your diet also can lower your blood pressure.

Healthy Weight

Being overweight or obese increases your risk for stroke. To determine whether your weight is in a healthy range, doctors often calculate your body mass index (BMI). If you know your weight and height, you can calculate your BMI at CDC's Assessing Your Weight Web site. Doctors sometimes also use waist and hip measurements to measure excess body fat.

Physical Activity

Physical activity can help you maintain a healthy weight and lower your cholesterol and blood pressure levels. For adults, the Surgeon General recommends 2 hours and 30 minutes of moderate-intensity exercise, like brisk walking or bicycling, every week. Children and adolescents should get 1 hour of physical activity every day.

No Smoking

Cigarette smoking greatly increases your risk for stroke. If you don't smoke, don't start. If you do smoke, quitting will lower your risk for stroke. Your doctor can suggest ways to help you quit.

Limited Alcohol

Avoid drinking too much alcohol, which can raise your blood pressure. Men should have no more than 2 drinks per day, and women only 1.

This previous section:

*Some Stroke Facts of Life* is compliments of the:

Centers for Disease Control (CDC) website.

# APPENDIX IV

# THE GAME-CHANGERS – A LIST

*What is a Game-Changer to me?*

Throughout the 44 chapters of this book I have tried to identify strategies and actions that I, we discovered during our journey. Some occurred after much effort, others, less so and some really by fortune or accident. But each made a difference to my recovery and/or our lifestyle going forward. So I called them Game-Changers because each in their own way changed the game to the positive. I have tried to discuss each of them in the context of a story. This is a personal and holistic list. We are all so different and individual, so we, each, could have a different set of Game-Changers. But I thought as part of the book it would be helpful to share my list in summary fashion.

**I would be interested in others' ideas, others' experiences, others' Game-Changers. Perhaps I can learn from you. We are all a community! – Please email me at <u>bob@strokevictor.com</u>.**

Chapter(s)

1. Let 911 do their thing.     2
2. Take your own reading material to the Doctor's office or hospital to avoid infection     26
3. As fast as possible, create a lifestyle that is as close as possible to normal.     5, 13
4. Surprise -It's easier to go up hills and stairs than down after a disability.     5
5. When you can't do something, think coping strategies to achieve your task.     Book
6. Understand, it's one thing to do a task while being supervised, and quite another to do it, unsupervised, particularly in a different location – don't panic!     6, 7

# WE ALL CAN BE STROKE VICTORS!

CPSIA information can be obtained
at www.ICGtesting.com
Printed in the USA
BVHW050904310721
612915BV00003B/227